Profile of the Negro in American Dentistry

PROFILE

OF THE NEGRO

IN AMERICAN

DENTISTRY

Edited by
Foster Kidd, D.D.S.

*and prepared under
the supervision of the
Society for Research and Study
of the Negro in Dentistry, Inc.*

HOWARD UNIVERSITY PRESS   *Washington, D.C. 1979*

Library of Congress Cataloging in Publication Data

Profile of the Negro in American dentistry.

   Bibliography: p.
   Includes index.
   1. Negroes in dentistry.   2. Dentistry—United
States—History. I. Kidd, Foster, 1924-
II. Society for Research and Study of the Negro in
Dentistry. [DNLM: 1. Dentistry—History—United
States. 2. Negroes—History—United States. WU11 AA1 P9]
RK34.U6P76   301.44'46   79–16159
ISBN 9-88258-034-5

Acknowledgments

The authors are obligated to a large number of people who aided and encouraged us throughout this project. Among them are Dr. Clifton O. Dummett, editor, *The Quarterly* of the National Dental Association, who was most kind in making available back issues of that journal and other documents; Dr. E. N. Jackson, NDA executive secretary, who made available the records, information, and copies of the Association's minutes we requested; also Drs. Eugenia Mobley, Jeanne Sinkford, Mary Jane Watkins, Juliann Bluitt, and Mrs. Allene Wallace, without whose help Chapter V, "Women in Dentistry" could not have been completed.

We are deeply indebted to Dr. R. B. Taylor, Sr., NDA Chaplain, for his untiring efforts in collecting data on Oklahoma dentists and information on the widows of deceased past presidents of the NDA. We are also grateful to Dr. E. H. Browne for his information on Texas dentists and for his inspiration throughout the project.

Many dentists throughout the United States responded to our query on the number of black dentists in their respective states, and also took their valuable time to complete and return our questionnaire. To them we also owe a debt of gratitude.

There were numerous persons outside the profession who helped with the production of this book: Herman P. Miller, chief, Population Division, Bureau of the Census; Naomi Lede, coordinator, Urban Research Center, Texas Southern University, Annette Flowers, department of business, Bishop College; C. B.

Bunkley, Jr., legal counsel, and Irving Baker, assistant to the president and director of Black Studies programs, Southern Methodist University (SMU); Opal Jones and, Geraldine Flowers, typists; and Ann Pence Davis, instructor, creative writing, SMU, who worked very diligently with the editor throughout his attendance in her classes.

We are also very grateful to Dr. Milton Curry, president of Bishop College, for allowing us to store our documents in the College library vaults; Cordie Hines, assistant chief of Branch Services, Dallas Public Library, for reviewing the manuscript, Eula Oliphant and Edward Hardge, librarians, Forest Avenue Branch, Dallas Public Library, for their invaluable aid in locating reference books.

We are obligated to the Board of Trustees of the NDA for their vote of approval of the project and to the entire leadership and membership of the NDA for their tolerance and patience.

I am indebted to my wife, Pearl Kidd, who reviewed the draft and constantly encouraged me to continue, and to my daughters, Cheryl and Tina, who toiled many long evenings with the surveys, charts, and mailings. For their support and understanding, I owe more than I can repay.

The authors would also like to thank the management and staff of the Howard University Press, particularly Charles F. Harris and Shirlene D. Evans, whose thoughts and guidance are reflected throughout the book.

To all of these persons and many more, the officers and members of the Society for Research and Study of the Negro in Dentistry, Inc., are eternally grateful.

Foster Kidd, D.D.S

Preface

The profession of dentistry has undergone many radical changes in the 1970s. The new format calls for all practitioners to prevent the occurrence and progression of dental disease and to search for oral pathological changes that may be the initial symptoms of systemic diseases. More professionals are needed to attend to the massive increase in health care services required by the inner city, as the profession moves ahead with increasing speed in the area of prevention, a whole new concept of oral health care. A greater number of personnel will be needed in teaching, research, and the administration of health programs on a group basis. The total number of blacks in the profession is insufficient to meet these new demands.

On a national basis, the ratio is one black dentist to every 12,500 blacks; in some areas the ratio is one-to-40,000. The general dentist-to-population ratio is one-to-2,000, and in a few states, the ratio is one-to-1,200 or one-to-1,400 people. (It has been suggested that ratios in this range *should* be available to the population nationwide.)

Approximately 3,200 new dentists graduate each year. Of this number, about 2,400 are needed annually to replace the dentists who die or retire. Most of the remaining 800 new dentists enter private practice. This figure sounds impressive, but it pales beside the realization that the national population increases by approximately three million each year, a ratio of new dentists to new population of one to approximately 4,000. Compare this to the one-to-2,000 ratio that we now have, and it follows that more dentists must be graduated to alleviate this critical situation.

The decade of the 1970s also has begun to usher in many innovative programs for motivating, identifying, and recruiting blacks to enter the profession. These plans should be welcomed by all, especially in view of the limited knowledge of predental requirements shown by some advisors, teachers, and counselors.

The scarcity of written material on the black dentist is another factor contributing to the lack of interest in the profession. Young blacks simply do not know enough about dentistry, less about the role of blacks within it, and nothing at all about their contributions to it.

Members of the dental profession have the duty to fill this void in raising public awareness of the contributions of the black dentist to society. Concerned persons have the responsibility to develop a new understanding of dentral care in the "new day in health" and to recruit more blacks into the field.

This book was written to serve this need. *Profile of the Negro in American Dentistry* is intended not only to point up the significant contributions of black dentists, but also to provide students, counselors, reseachers, and concerned individuals with valuable material about the dental profession as a whole. Emphasis is placed on every aspect, from dental schools to dental organizations, scholarship and loan sources, manufacturers, suppliers, laboratories, and professional and technical personnel.

Contents

Profile of the Negro in American Dentistry

Introduction

Dentistry, as we know it today, was not practiced in America until the middle of the nineteenth century, although as early as 1697 the French had begun to establish rules for its practice. Any man who wished to enroll in the College of Surgeons, work for two years with a licensed dentist, pass an examination on the theory and practice of dentistry, and take an oath before the Chief Surgeon could be licensed to practice in France. However, most of the licensed dentists serviced only the wealthy, while barber surgeons, tooth drawers, and itinerant charlatans served the general public.

In Colonial America, the influence of French dentistry was seen in the early techniques and instruments used by all recognized practitioners. As in France, there were also barbers, blacksmiths, itinerant quacks—and even jewelers—who functioned as dentists.

The first recorded reference to a black practitioner of dentistry in America was in 1740, a man called Simon, "who was regarded as being able to bleed and draw teeth, and . . . pretended to be a great doctor among his people."[1] By 1840 the number of blacks practicing dentistry was estimated to be 120; all had been apprentices and laboratorians to white dentists.

Prior to their arrival in America, Africans rarely experienced diseases of the oral cavity such as periodontal diseases and dental caries (decay of bone or tooth). Those periodontal disturbances that had been observed were due primarily to the

African's native custom of sharpening and decorating his teeth, rather than to disease. However, after being transported to the New World and subjected to dietary changes, slaves showed a gradual increase in dental caries.

The greatest occurrence of dental caries was among the house servants who ate the same foods as their masters and mistresses. On the other hand, field slaves experienced little increase in caries, because they ate produce of the fields and continued to prepare meals in a manner similar to their native custom. When medical or dental problems did develop, the field hands, for the most part, had to provide their own curative methods, while house servants were usually treated by the family physician.

Few slave children enjoyed a nutritious diet that helped to produce good teeth or received dental attention and, as a result, they often suffered from tooth decay as adults. Consequently, the image of the plantation black with a broad grin and glistening teeth—so popular in early white literature—is more fiction than fact. A very large proportion of the advertisements for fugitive slaves described their teeth as "much rotten" or "somewhat decayed."

Because of the lack of professional dental care, the majority of slaves not only developed new procedures in caring for their teeth but also continued to use techniques carried over from Africa. The Makatese tribe of West Africa, for example, extracted a child's tooth by tying it to a strong, thin sinew attached to the spoke of an ox wagon wheel. A piece of iron was heated and suddenly thrust close to the face of the child who, forgetting his tooth and thinking only of the danger in front of him, jerked away. The early generation of slaves in Virginia continued this custom by tying one end of a strong cord to a child's tooth and the other to a doorknob. The tooth was extracted when the door was opened unexpectedly.

According to Dr. Ford Johnson of Martinsville, Virginia, the gold open-face or full crown had its origin in Africa, where human teeth were an important part of tribal life and objects of severe measure during tribal initiations and ceremonies. This belief in the importance of teeth continued in America, where the crown became an award, bestowed mostly upon children, on a special occasion such as graduation from elementary or high school, or a birthday.

Until the fourth decade of the nineteenth century, there had been few changes in dental practice for some two hundred years. Teeth were neglected until they fell out or were pulled. Toothache was treated by local applications or by extractions, and physicians were called upon for both. In general, it might be stated that before 1830, many itinerant practitioners were blatant quacks, although some were unquestionably well-trained and competent for that time.

Despite the public need and demand for competent dentists and professional dental care, itinerant charlatans continued to multiply. Their numbers increased in such alarming proportions that it became mandatory to create cohesive restrictions for the protection of the public and the profession. Legislation was proposed and medical and dental societies were founded with the aim of elevating the quality of the profession and protecting citizens from impositions practiced upon them by unprincipled itinerants.

Recognized dentists were predominantly white and viewed with disdain the task of providing dental care to free blacks. Many dentists refused to threat Negroes; some dentists accepted black patients only in the evening after closing hours or early in the morning before opening. Negroes were also required to use the back stairs and to wait in isolated areas designated especially for them.

Eventually, more blacks began to enter dentistry, primarily because of their awareness that this move afforded them the opportunity to hold professional positions and to rise above their former menial status before the Civil War. By the end of the War, large numbers of Negroes distinguished themselves in the field. Dental education had become somewhat standardized, and preparation for a career in the field had risen from an apprenticeship to dental college attendance. Blacks, however, were denied admission to dental schools until Harvard University admitted Robert Tanner Freeman, the first black to graduate (in 1867). Subsequently, many northern schools opened their doors to blacks on a quota basis. By 1890 Howard University College of Dentistry and Meharry Medical College School of Dentistry had graduated several classes of university-trained dentists, and by 1900 there were 125 Negro dentists practicing in the United States.

Though discrimination by local, state, and national medical societies was widespread, early black dentists made significant contributions to the profession in spite of being denied easy access to new discoveries and information. Charles Edwin Bentley (a graduate of the Chicago College of Dental Surgery in 1887), for example, initiated programs that served as the blueprint for educational institutions throughout America. He was the founder and first president of the Odontographic Society of Chicago. Dr. Bentley was, perhaps, best known as the father of the oral hygiene movement, and for instituting dental examinations in public schools. He was also the first dentist in Chicago to use cocaine as an anesthetic and the first oral surgeon of the newly established Provident Hospital under the leadership of Daniel Hale Williams.

Many early black dentists tried to break down racial barriers through social and political action; others, by training blacks in various phases of dentistry. A Cincinnati, Ohio dentist, Ellard Cox, was active in the training of black dental technicians. His former pupil, Joseph Hurst, opened the first black dental laboratory in that city in 1944.

Through the efforts of black dental organizations, social, political, and professional barriers have been effectively confronted—particularly through the National Dental Association (NDA), which represents almost 2,000 black dentists in America. Founded in the early 1900s, this organization serves poverty and ghetto areas. Its constitution specifically states that it will, among other things, "work persistently for the elimination of religious and racial discrimination, and segregation from American dental institutions, clinics, and organizations."

In 1969, under the chairmanship of Harvey Webb, Jr., the

legislative committee of the NDA presented a statement of its Board of Trustees criticizing the dental establishment for neglecting the poor and the federal government for its handling of dental-care programs:

> From past experience we cannot assume that the dental profession as we know it and as represented by the American Dental Association acts in the best interest of the poor consumer. Often only the vested interests are served by the American Dental Association. We know that the American Dental Association refuses to represent that segment of the population charged with the responsibility of providing care to the nearly twenty-five million Blacks in the country. . . . We submit that on the basis of past performance, the Department of Health, Education and Welfare in general, the Division of Dental Health and bodies appointed to supervise the equitable administration of Federal dental-care programs, have left much to be desired and that the NDA can no longer afford to stand by and observe injustices perpetrated against the poor and the Black people of this country.

Service to the black community has always been stressed by Meharry and Howard, the two schools that graduate the majority of black dentists. Both schools have created substantial dental-care programs in the communities they serve, and Howard annually transports hundreds of children from rural Mississippi to provide them with dental treatment and other health services. Both schools are constantly revising their curricula and updating their facilities, so that graduates may learn to serve the black community more efficiently.

In 1960, there were 81,249 dentists employed in the United States. Of this number, 78,370 were white and 1,998 were black. The number of black dentists has fluctuated rather curiously during the past forty years. In 1939, for example, there were 1,773 black dentists. Twenty years later, the number had shrunk

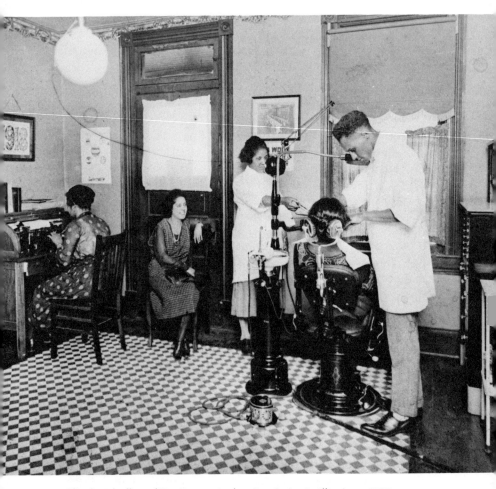

The dental office of Dr. Monroe Jordan, East St. Louis, Illinois, c. 1919.

to 1,681. From 1960 to 1970, their number continued to rise to
the present 2,206-plus. The ratio of black dentists to the black
population has remained constant at 1-to-12,500, while the
national dentist-population ratio improves (in 1969, it was
1-to-1,693). But some observers maintain that this is true be-

cause fifty percent of all black dentists practice in fifteen metropolitan areas (see Appendix D).

For whatever reason, more black dentists, as well as other dental personnel, are urgently needed to provide quality health care to the public. Not only general practitioners but specialists, researchers, teachers, hygienists, technicians, and dental assistants are also needed.

Chapter I

Black Pioneers in American

Dentistry

Early Black Dentists in Virginia

Before 1830 dentistry in Virginia (and elsewhere) could be practiced by anyone who called himself a dentist. Because the dental schools were not responding rapidly enough to the public need and demand for dentists, itinerant practitioners—both the quacks and the competent—soon began to grow in number. It became apparent that, for the protection of the public and the reputation of the dental profession, more stringent restrictions would have to be imposed. It also became mandatory to recognize the qualified, established, practitioners who lacked the degree but who, by professional achievement, were worthy of inclusion in the profession.

Finally, in 1842, the Virginia Society of Surgeons and Dentists was founded and immediately began to press for new legislation and the enforcement of existing laws. Excluded from this society, of course, were blacks. However, after the Civil War Negroes began to practice dentistry in increasing numbers. Unlike white dentists, most blacks of the post-Civil War period did not have sufficient finances to equip and open dental offices. Consequently, this group (who became known as "street dentists") carried instruments with them and performed services in the streets or in patients' homes. According to Dr. Stephen Lewis of Manassas, street dentists received their training from whites for whom they had worked as office helpers or body servants during the Civil War. After the War, black dentists began their own practices, drawing patients from among the Negroes whom the whites were reluctant to treat.

Two outstanding and very proficient early street dentists were Charles B. Jackson and John Christian (both of Richmond), who practiced from 1883 to 1902. These men took pride in their profession and distinguished themselves by wearing long-tailed black frock coats and high hats.

However, such concern and ability did not characterize all who called themselves dentists; charlatans also thrived. Peter Hawkins—one of the most colorful—operated from an office that boasted the shingle, THE HOUSE OF PETER HAWKINS, TOOTH DRAWER. A tall, gaunt, very black man, Hawkins rode about the streets on a rawboned black horse, carrying two or three pullikins in his pockets. One of his former patients, Samuel Mordecai, recalled seeing a man who was writhing in agony stop Hawkins in the street and plead for an immediate extraction. Hawkins quickly reached for his pullikins and deftly relieved his patient, without dismounting from his horse. The great strength in his wrist could mean trouble for his patients: while extracting an offending tooth, he would inevitably break or extract other sound teeth in the immediate area!

Another itinerant dentist, A.C.S. Robinson, a sign painter by trade, lived in Suffolk during the 1920s. According to Dr. James Colden of the area, Robinson made gold crowns and placed diamonds in his patients' teeth. He continued this practice after the State Dental Board began to enforce its qualifications. Eventually, Robinson was called into court for failing to obtain a license to practice dentistry.

Still another practitioner, Mrs. Perkins of Stafford County, performed early extractions. It was a common practice of the time for citizens to extract their neighbors' teeth by using ordinary household pliers, according to Dr. Calloway Wyatt of Richmond. If the roots broke off, they were left in the sockets. (This practice existed as late as 1900.)

Custom and superstition continued to guide dental practice. in many areas of Virginia, despite the continuous upgrading of the profession and the availability of more competent dentists. A favorite treatment among both blacks and whites was the use of bluestone, a vitriol which killed the nerve and turned the tooth blue-black. In some areas, people would permit extractions only if the signs of the zodiac were favorable.

Although the majority of the black practitioners of the post-Civil War period were street dentists, Thomas Bayne of Norfolk was able to maintain regular offices. Born a slave in 1823, Dr. Bayne escaped to England and later returned as a free man to Boston, where he acquired the equivalent of a secondary education and studied dentistry. His penchant for the political arena soon caused him to return to Norfolk, where he entered politics and began a dental practice. Dr. Bayne was one of Norfolk's two representatives to the Constitutional Convention of 1867-68, where he became known for his struggle against racial discrimination in Virginia schools.

In spite of the fact that little emphasis was placed on preparing young people for the profession before 1839, Horace Hayden of Baltimore finally succeeded in establishing a course in dentistry at the University of Maryland during the years 1837-38. The tremendous opposition from medical doctors spurred Dr. Hayden to establish the Baltimore College of Dental Surgery in 1839, the first official dental school in the world. In subsequent years other schools opened: Howard University College of Dentistry (1881), Meharry Dental School (1886), and Virginia Medical College of Dentistry (1893). In 1859 the American Dental Association (ADA) was formed to create standard policies of operation and to formulate guidelines for setting uniform standards for dental graduates.

This national concern for establishing and maintaining quality dentistry manifested itself in the passing of the Virginia State Board of Dental Examiners Act on November 6, 1886. Meeting in Richmond at Ford's Hotel, the Board made it unlawful for anyone except an authorized physician or surgeon to engage in the practice of dentistry or to receive a license as a dentist from any commissioner of revenue, unless the person had received a diploma from a reputable institution or had obtained a certificate from the Board of Examiners the Act created. (Nothing in this Act, however, prevented laymen from extracting teeth.) The Act also stipulated that its provisions should not apply to persons engaged in the practice of dentistry on or before February 28, 1886.

Charles B. Jackson, the early street dentist, was the first black dentist to be licensed in Virginia; he registered with the Board in 1886. His colleague, John Christian, failed to register even after laws passed in 1900 required all practitioners to do so. Thus, Dr. Christian was forced to discontinue his practice. The first black to receive a certificate from the Board was Peter B. Ramsey, a Meharry graduate, for whom the local dental societies of Petersburg and Richmond are named. Another pioneering black dentist was David A. Ferguson, the first black to take the State Board's written examination in 1900.

The beginning of the twentieth century saw an appreciable rise in the number of black men entering the field of dentistry. White practitioners, although sensitive to their white patients' prejudices against blacks who shared the profession, encouraged skilled office assistants, who were already competent and knowledgeable in dental techniques, to attend either Meharry or Howard dental schools at the expense of their employers.

William T. Lovett of Norfolk began his career in such a manner. He was noticed in the streets by Millison Allen, a white physician, who hired Lovett to serve as his office orderly and hack driver. Noticing undeveloped potential in Lovett, Dr. Allen sent the young black to Howard University's College of Dentistry during the early part of the twentieth century. Upon completion of his training in 1903, Lovett returned to Norfolk, took the State Board exam, and became a licensed dentist.

From 1903 to 1913, many other blacks passed the State Board and established practices throughout Virginia, including T. A. Stevens (1903), the first black dentist in Lynchburg, W. W. Jackson (1906), who followed Dr. Lovett to Norfolk, and J. G. Ramsey (1907) of Richmond.

TABLE 1

BLACK DENTISTS IN VIRGINIA, 1903-13

Name	City	Date of State Board
W. T. Lovett	Norfolk	1903
T. A. Stevens	Lynchburg	1903
Wesley W. Jefferson	Norfolk	1906
J. M. G. Ramsey	Richmond	1907
F. P. Barrier	Alexandria	1907
Roscoe Brown	Richmond	1907
John L. McGriff	Portsmouth	1908
E. R. Dudley	Roanoke	1909
Norman Lassiter	Newport News	1909
O. W. Marshall	Staunton	1909
J. T. Lattimore	Newport News	1909
J. E. Geary	Danville	1909
J. H. Haskins	Appalachia	1911
George C. Strong	Norfolk	1911
E. L. H. Rance	Suffolk	1911
W. B. Anderson	Portsmouth	1912
O. R. Johnson	Petersburg	1912
E. D. Downing	Roanoke	1913
F. S. Coppage	Norfolk	1913
R. J. Brown	Norfolk	1913

Source: City directories of Norfolk, Postsmouth, and Berkley, Virginia, 1897, 1898, 1899, 1900, and 1902.

Early Black Dentists in Ohio

Perhaps the most striking figure to emerge in black dentistry from Ohio was Reginald Beamon of Cincinnati, who contributed vastly to the professional, social, and political advancement of blacks in that city. Virginia-born, a graduate of Howard University's liberal arts and dental colleges and dental officer in World War I, Dr. Beamon began his practice around the turn of the twentieth century.

A large man with an engaging manner, Dr. Beamon is remembered by friends and colleagues for his constantly pleasant demeanor under depressing circumstances. He personally encouraged and recruited blacks to settle in Cincinnati, opened his office to them, and made available his personal resources to further their careers in the profession.

Beamon ran as the first black candidate for councilman on the Charter Party ticket, even though the Republican Party had urged him to run as their candidate and assured him of victory. He believed strongly that the corrupt political machine and Saturday-night paternalism, then rife in Cincinnati, were detrimental to the black community.

One incident illustrates Beamon's firm stand against racial discrimination. The Charter Party met in the old Sinton Hotel—the epitome of elegance in the city—which prohibited blacks from entering or using any of the facilities. When blacks were seated in the balcony of the ballroom for a Charter meeting and dinner, Beamon voiced his displeasure and left, despite the entreaties of the Mayor. He repeated this performance on another occasion, until barriers were broken down and all Charter members—black and white—were seated together on the main floor.

Recognizing the need for an organization to exert pressure in changing existing dental practices and to bring black dentists into the mainstream, Dr. Beamon helped to organize the Molar Club in 1929 (which became the Ohio Valley Dental Society in 1934). The Society adopted the following proposals:

1. to improve techniques and practices;
2. to insure high ethics among members;
3. to band together in a common goal against dentists who advertised;
4. to use a political base from which to fight for membership in the Cincinnati Dental Society.

During the period, in Cincinnati, the practice of dentistry abounded with white dentists who advertised their services primarily to blacks and poor whites. Because of this odious situation caused by the neglect of the Cincinnati Dental Society, the Molar Club urged a black state legislator on the health committee to petition the legislature for action. The results of their efforts brought about the following regulations:

1. Only licensed dentists were permitted to open a dental office.

2. Licensed dentists were required to be graduates of an accredited dental school.

2. Dentists were forbidden to advertise fees.

4. Specific regulations were adopted for passing the state dental examination.

For their efforts on behalf of organized dentistry (with the assistance of sympathetic white dentists, who recognized the contribution of Dr. Beamon and others) the members of the Molar Club were granted membership in the Cincinnati Dental Society and ultimately the ADA.

Pioneering dentists like Beamon helped to raise the standards of dentistry among blacks and created order from chaos. Their counterparts today face many of the same problems that plagued these earlier dentists. Though much progress has been made in every aspect of the profession, much remains to be accomplished before blacks can consider themselves part of the mainstream of American dentistry.

Chapter II

Black Dental Schools

Howard University College of Dentistry
Washington, D.C.

The Howard University College of Dentistry began October 11, 1881, with the appointment of James B. Hodgkin as lecturer on practical dentistry to the medical class. The appointment was made in recognition of the need for physicians practicing in remote areas to also provide dental care.

The first permanent professor of dentistry, N.W. Whitcomb, was appointed on June 5, 1882. However, it was not until 1883-84 that the first regular course in dentistry began. Matriculation was open to anyone who qualified for the medical college.[1] Candidates for graduation were required to be at least twenty-one years of age, to attend two years of lectures at a regular dental college (at least one at Howard) or, in lieu of one year of college, to have spent five years in dental practice. In addition, candidates must comply with all regulations concerning lectures, dissections, and mecanical work to the satisfaction of staff.

Five students completed the first year's course of study and one satisfied the requirements for graduation. The second year, the College produced another graduate and several additions to the faculty, although Dr. Whitcomb, its first appointed professor, resigned because of other commitments and lack of sufficient financial support for the new College. Starr Parsons was appointed professor of dental surgery and operative dentistry, William Leitch, a Howard graduate, was appointed to teach operative and prosthetic dentistry. In addition, two other dentists were named clinical instructors.

In its third year, the faculty made additional changes that strengthened the basic curriculum. Students were required to treat actual patients and to submit their treatment plans to the professor of operative dentistry, to prepare artificial dentures, and to provide an artificial replacement for at least one approved patient. In addition to the standard examinations, candidates for graduation were required to submit a thesis on a subject related to dentistry.

On April 23, 1890, the first Dean of the College of Dentistry was elected by the faculty. He was J.F.R. Dufour, a highly respected member of the Medical School staff. With Dr. Dufour's selection, a reorganization of the College of Dentistry began, during which time, the curriculum was constantly improved and broadened to encompass the medical sciences and to provide rational treatment planning, clinical demonstration, and practice.

Another administrative reorganization occurred in 1896, at which time the office of Dean of the College of Dentistry was abolished. A new office of Dean of the Medical School—which included the dental and pharmaceutical colleges—was created. Administrative refinements continued until 1904, when the vice-Dean of the Medical School, Andrew Brown, an 1890 graduate of the College, was placed in charge of dentistry.

The dental college continued to grow and prosper to such an extent that by 1907-08 there were 6 graduates from a student body of 58, and between the years 1901 and 1910, a total of 115 graduates. In 1909 the academic year was increased to 32 weeks of six days each; by 1917 the curriculum increased from two years to four years of study. In addition, students were no longer permitted to substitute five years of practical experience for one year of study.

The economic depression that began in the late 1920s, along

with the relatively high cost of dental education, caused a decline in enrollments. The increasingly visible needs of a poor and segregated black population, coupled with the College's attempt to elevate the standard of dental education in the face of a declining student body, posed serious problems for the administrative and faculty. Faced with a Class B rating due, in part, to an inadequate physical plant, the Dean and faculty of the College of Dentistry began to undertake a total reorganization of both faculty and curriculum, as well as an upgrading of the facilities.

A new School of Medicine was established in 1929, incorporating the colleges of medicine, dentistry, and pharmacy. Each college was independently administered by its own dean and faculty. Under this plan, Arnold Donawa (a Howard College of Dentistry graduate) became the first academic dean of the College of Dentistry. He was succeeded by Russell A. Dixon, who was appointed acting dean in 1931 and Dean in 1934.[2] And in 1943—nearly ten years after Dr. Dixon's appointment—the Council on Dental Education of the ADA granted the College a provisional acceptable rating. In 1948 the Council awarded the College full accreditation in Class A. Dr. Dixon served as dean until 1966, when Joseph L. Henry was appointed to that position. On July 1, 1975 Jeanne Sinkford was appointed dean of the university's College of Dentistry. Dr. Sinkford was the first woman to be appointed dean of any dental school in the nation.

Since the mid-sixties, the College has continued to improve its physical facilities as well as reorganize its educational programs to produce competent practitioners in the art and science of dentistry. Its commitment to excellence has remained constant, with a number of significant innovations and improvements, including the advancement of a strong recruitment program for black students and faculty and the establishment of an academic reinforcement program to improve the performance of all students; initiation of programs designed to teach and deliver dental treatment to the chronically ill and aged on an out-patient basis; revision of the curriculum to include the correlated course concept, reducing classroom lecture time without affecting course emphasis or teaching effectiveness; establishment of multidisciplinary clinical-laboratory facilities; initiation of four-handed multiple-operatory practice concepts; training in dental hygiene, to include functions usually performed by a licensed dentist; establishment of graduate programs in orthodontics, oral surgery, and pedodontics; establishment of the Department of Hospital Dentistry and an increase in research programs; and most notably, establishment of the National Institutes of Health Adolescent-Periodontal Research Unit.

Howard University's recruitment program is one of the most sophisticated in the country, costing approximately $25,000 annually, a budget which includes the visits of representatives to black colleges, conferences with local counselors and civic organizations, predental study clubs on other college campuses, high-school level recruitment, and distribution of special brochures and displays at local and national meetings.

Meharry Medical College School of Dentistry
Nashville, Tennessee

In 1876 the institution that was to become Meharry Medical College was part of the Medical Department of Central Tennessee College, an institution founded by the Freedman's Aid Society of the Methodist Episcopal Church in 1866. The College was named for the Meharry family, the members of which liberally contributed to its establishment and early support.

The first classes of the Medical Department were held in 1866 in the basement of Clark Memorial Church, just one year after the Civil War. George W. Hubbard, a medical corpsman in the Union Army, was the first dean. Assisting Dr. Hubbard was a former surgeon of the Confederate Army, W.G. Sneed.

During the 1880s, medical graduates of Meharry felt the need for a dental facility. In addition to the model provided by the Vanderbilt School of Dentistry in Nashville, there were many professionals who held both dental and medical degrees. One such person, William Henry Morgan (dean of the Vanderbilt School), helped to establish the dental school at Meharry.

In 1886, Meharry Medical College School of Dentistry began as the Department of Dentistry of Central Tennessee College (which was incorporated into Walden University in 1900) and remained so until 1915, at which time Meharry was granted a separate charter by the State of Tennessee.

The first session of the School of Dentistry began on October 4, 1886, and continued for twenty weeks. J. P. Bailey, the first dean of Meharry's dental facility and an 1881 graduate of Vanderbilt, taught operative and mechanical dentistry. Dean Morgan of Vanderbilt lectured and demonstrated in the clinic, as did several local dentists. The first group of students included three medical school graduates (J. W. Anderson, R. F. Boyd, and H. T. Noel) and six others who did not hold medical degrees.

The curriculum encompassed two years of study. The first year included anatomy, chemistry, and physiology, along with practical work in the dental infirmary and laboratory. During the second year, students studied advanced anatomy (including dissection), along with dental hygience and *materia medica*. Additional hours were spent in the laboratory and infirmary. Reference works, at that time, were limited to John Tomes's *Dental Surgery*, Jonathan Taft's *Operative Dentistry*, Joseph Richardson's *Mechanical Dentistry*, and E. Wildman's *Instruction in Vulcanite Work*.

Tuition was thirty dollars per year, and the graduation fee was ten dollars. Instructional materials were furnished at cost. Personal expenses—room, board, fuel, lights and laundry—amounted to nine or ten dollars a month, depending upon the needs of the individual student.

During this era, medical and dental credits were given equal evaluation, and graduates of the school could graduate from Meharry Medical Department by attending one session and passing the required examination. Three medical graduates completed the dental course in one year to become the Class of 1887, the first to graduate from the School of Dentistry.

In 1890 Dean Bailey entered private practice, and two years later J. B. Singleton, Sr. (an 1892 graduate of Meharry) became director of the school. Dr. Singleton retired in 1921, and was replaced by D. H. Turpin, a graduate of the Class of 1918, also a Meharry faculty member, and staff dentist at the George W. Hubbard Hospital.

During the Great Depression of the 1930s, dental schools declined; student enrollment dropped, and competent teachers could not be retained. Some thought that the Meharry School of Dentistry would join the other dental institutions in closing. However, in 1938, E. L. Turner succeeded J. J. Mullowney as President and began to reestablish various departments in the School of Medicine and Dentistry. He named Dr. Turpin Dean of the School of Dentistry, and in 1942 persuaded M. Don Clawson, a former colleague at the American University in Beirut, Lebanon, to join the faculty as Director of dental education. Also during this time, Clifton O. Dummett joined the faculty as instructor in peridontics. Under Dr. Clawson's guidance, the School of Dentistry began to receive financial aid of considerable magnitude—the Kellogg Foundation support was especially noteworthy. Dr. Clawson and Dr. Turpin also worked closely together in reorganizing the curriculum.

In 1945 Dr. Clawson was elected President of Meharry Medical College, and Dr. Turpin served as dean until his death in 1947.* William H. Allen, already a member of the faculty and Chairman of the Department of Prosthodontics, was named Dean of the School of Dentistry in 1949. President Clawson, on sabbatical leave, was elected to the Board of Trustees in 1950, and from 1950 to 1952, the affairs of the Medical College were administered by an interim committee. In 1952 the trustees elected the first black president of Meharry, Harold D. West, who for twenty-five years was Associate Professor of Biochemistry at the College.

In 1969 Lloyd Elam, director of the department of psychiatry and acting dean, was elected president of the Medical College. Two years later, after Dean Allen's retirement, Thomas P. Logan was named dean of the School of Dentistry.**

---

*Dr. Clifton O. Dummett was appointed dean in 1947, a post held until he resigned in 1949.

** Logan served as dean until 1978, and was succeeded by Eugenia Mobley, the first woman dean of Meharry and is one of only two female deans in the United States.

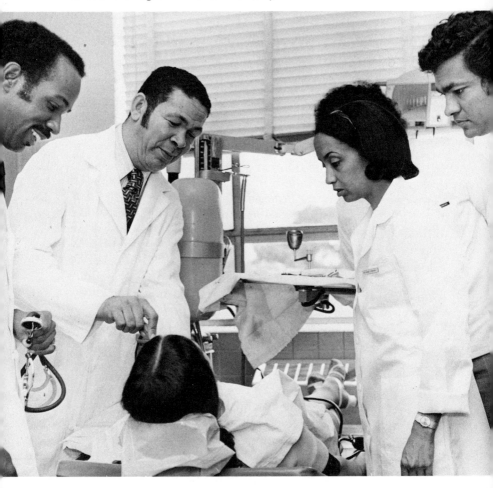

Dr. Jeanne Sinkford (second from right), dean of Howard University College of Dentistry, and Dr. Joseph L. Henry (second from left), former dean, discuss patient's problem with students.

The Division of Dental Hygiene at Meharry Medical College was organized as an integral part of the School of Dentistry in 1931. Until 1940, the Division awarded diplomas upon completion of one year of dental hygiene, preceded by one year of dental practice training. In September of 1944 the Division was reorganized under its present two-year curriculum and fully accredited by the Council on Dental Education of the ADA. Its graduates are eligible for license examinations in all states and territories of the United States.

Traditionally, the number of Dental Hygiene matriculants had been limited in order to provide superior laboratory, classroom, and clinical work for each individual commensurate with the professional staff and facilities. Presently, innovative programs—some experimental in nature—are being planned so that more qualified young people can study at Meharry. These prorams would also enable the Division of Dental Hygiene to continue its role in providing optimal dental care for all citizens.

Meharry Medical College School of Dentistry, like the Howard University College of Dentistry, has taken on new dimensions in recent years: renovation of its physical plant; installment of additional dental units as a result of government special project grant funds; revision of the curriculum to include preventive dentistry; and recruitment of additional faculty and staff members in continuing its commitment to excellence. The recruitment committee conducts a series of tours for visiting students to encourage potential applicants. Meharry has also developed a program in which college students, science teachers, premedical/predental advisors, high school teachers, and guidance counselors attend orientation programs in the fields of medicine and dentistry at Meharry.

Chapter III

The Dental Student

In January 1968 Foster Kidd surveyed 50 dental schools in the United States to ascertain the number of black students enrolled for the D.D.S. or D.M.D. degree. He found that blacks represented less than two percent of the total number. California, with 5 dental schools, had only 2 blacks and, with the exception of the Universities of Indiana and Puerto Rico (5 students each), no one dental school had more than 3 blacks.

Apparently, the situation had not changed since 1945 when Clifton O. Dummett, former dean of dental education at Meharry Medical College, noted a total of only 24 black students in 12 out of 37 predominantly white dental schools in the United States. (All other black students were enrolled at Howard or Meharry.) Dr. Dummett also observed that the number of black students in any one school did not exceed a total of 4. At that time there were 39 dental schools in this country, 12 of which had no black students and indicated that they would refuse to accept blacks.

In 1968, an editorial in the ADA *Journal* noted the scarcity of practicing black dentists but ignored the major cause of this situation. Russell A. Dixon, dean emeritus of Howard University College of Dentistry, wrote this response: "The editorial on Negro dental manpower in the January 1968 issue of the ADA *Journal* suggests a dilemma for dentistry which is foreboding and needs remedy. It gives no clear diagnosis of the ailments,

24

however, and offers no cure. . . ."[1]

Joseph L. Henry, former dean of the College of Dentistry at Howard University, also responded: "The time is ripe for all American dental schools to recruit and admit Negro students. This must include special efforts to identify students with ample potential . . . " He added, "It is my firm belief that the American Dental Association, the American Association of Dental Schools, and all organized dentistry have a great responsibility to recruit Negroes to dentistry as a part of their overall obligation to recruitment . . . "[2]

Howard and Meharry, the two dental schools in the United States that supply more than half of all black practitioners, graduate an average of 150 black men and women dentist annually. But other schools must increase their output of black dentists if the ever-widening gap of black dentists-to-black population ratio is to be improved. An increase in the enrollment of blacks in the nation's dental schools is apparent. Forty-five dental schools reported increased black enrollment during 1970-71, whereas only 37 schools enrolled black students in the 1969-70 academic year.

The failure of many dental schools to accept blacks is only one factor contributing to the shortage of black dentists. Other factors are lack of student motivation, lack of financial aid to students and guidance and counselling at the high school and college level, inadequate recruitment measures by the dental schools, and expanded employment opportunities for minority students in fields other than dentistry.

As organized dentistry responds to the need for increased dental personnel by motivating, identifying, and recruiting black students, these early barriers are being surmounted.

Financial aid is now possible for black dental students through a precedent-setting scholarship program begun in 1968 with a generous grant by the W.K. Kellogg Company to the American Fund for Dental Health (formerly the American Fund for Dental Education) of ADA. In 1970 there were 40 recipients of scholarships studying under this program. The long-range goal is to provide 265 scholarships per year, one for each class of

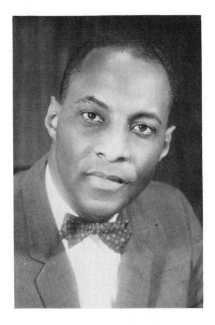

In 1947 Dr. Clifton O. Dummett was appointed dean of Meharry's school of dentistry, becoming at age 28 the youngest dental dean in the United States.

accredited dental schools and one for each predental class.

Frank E. Chowning, president of the NDA in 1968, originated a recruitment program entitled "Dentistry as a Career" and received a grant from the Coca Cola Company for its funding and implementation. Organizations participating in the Coca Cola program include Alpha Phi Alpha fraternity, the International Benevolent Protective Order of Elks (IBPOE), National Association for the Advancement of Colored People (NAACP), National Council of Negro Women, the NDA, National Medical Association (NMA), National Newspaper Publishers Association (NNPA), Omega Psi Phi fraternity, and the Ancient Egyptian Arabic Order Nobles of the Mystic Shrine (AEAONMS).

Meharry School of Dentistry and Howard University College of Dentistry scholarships are granted to sophomores, and loans are available to juniors and seniors. The two schools also participate in the Health Professions Education Assistance Act (HPEAA) through the Student Loan Act (see Appendix H).

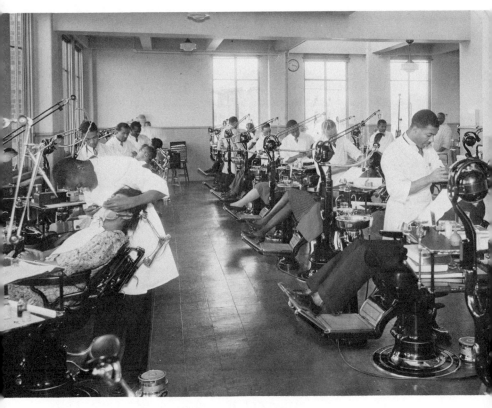

Students at work in early Meharry Patient Dental Clinic.

The average cost of a four-year dental education, exclusive of living costs, is approximately $15,000. Though this figure looms large in the minds of young college students, many plan their professional careers with considerable foresight. It is interesting to note that a number of students who do enter dental school have substantial personal savings available to meet all or part of school expenses. In addition to money received from parents and the students' personal saving, scholarships and loans, additional benefits are available to veterans of the Armed Services under the G.I. Bill of Rights.

Dental Aptitude Test

An ADA report (1968-70) stated that: "Performance of black students on the Dental Aptitude Test was below the national average in every subject. Nationally, predental students taking the test scored 3.75 in quantitative ability, 3.90 in reading ability, 4.0 in biology and chemistry, and 4.24 in manual dexterity. Black predental students scored 1.12 in quantitive ability, 1.74 in reading ability, 2.5 in biology and chemistry, and 2.58 in manual dexterity."

The shortcomings of black predental students on the Aptitude Test have not escaped the notice of educators. Maynard K. Hines, dean of the Indiana University Dental School, addressing a joint meeting of the NDA-ADA Liaison Committee on August 4, 1968, stated:

> . . . although there are exceptions, I think it is also true that in general, underprivileged students do not perform well [on] aptitude tests given by the American Dental Association. The aptitude test as it is now given depends in a great part on the past experience of the applicant. What is needed is a test to evaluate the potential of a student, and [based on] this potential, a placement test will be given to identify weaknesses alleviated by special courses in dental or predental school.

However, the Division of Educational Measurements of the ADA reported in a study covering the testing periods of October 1968 through January 1970, that the Dental Aptitude Test actually provides a much higher degree of accuracy in predicting the potential success of black students than of white students.

Student National Dental Association

The Student National Dental Association (SNDA) was established in 1972 as an organization committed to improving the status of minority dental students. As an affilate of the NDA the SNDA seeks to improve communication between minority dental students by disseminating a newsletter covering new developments within the dental profession, legislation affecting the practice, and current issues facing black dentists. The SNDA also gathers statistics and encourages Howard and Meharry students to join the organization before graduation.[3]

Chapter IV

Dental Specialties

The D.D.S. or D.M.D. degree qualifies the graduate of a recognized college of dentistry to treat all diseases of the oral cavity. Although the greatest percentage of black dentists engage in general practice, the number entering specialty fields is growing at a rapid pace.

Black specialties are found in the areas of oral surgery, orthodontics, pedodontics, and periodontics. There are also black endodontists, oral pathologists, public health dentists, and prosthodontists.

Approximately one of every eight dental school graduates accepts an internship and residency in a hospital. As a member of the house staff of a general or specialty hospital, the dentist receives advanced clinical experience, plus additional training in the sciences basic to dental practice. He or she also achieves proficiency in a specialized field of practice or research and the educational background for continued development in a special field. After two, or possibly three, years a dentist is examined by one of the national certifying boards recognized by the ADA.

The Eight Areas of Specialization Recognized
by the American Dental Association

Dental Public Health is that area of dentistry which seeks to prevent and control dental disease on a community level and promotes dental health through public education and organized community efforts.

Endodontics is devoted to treating infections of the pulp (nerve and blood vessels) of the tooth and the conditions that develop at the tip of the root as a result of infection.

Oral Pathology is concerned with the diagnosis of unusual diseases of the mouth which dental practitioners have discovered.

Oral Surgery deals with the diagnosis and the surgical and adjunctive treatment of diseases, injuries, and defects of the jaws and associated structures.

Orthodontics is concerned with the detection, study, prevention, and correction of irregularities in tooth position and jaw relationship, and of deformities of the face produced by these conditions.

Pedodontics is the dental equivalent of pediatrics in medicine. The pedodonist treats all oral health conditions in children, except those irregularities requiring major orthodontic treatment or surgery.

Periodontics is concerned with the diagnosis and treatment of diseases which affect the gums and other structures surrounding and supporting the teeth.

Prosthodontics involves the design and construction of dental appliances and substitutes for natural teeth, such as crowns, bridges, and dentures.

Dental Public Health

This specialty area seeks to prevent and control dental disease on a community level and promotes dental health through public education and organized community efforts. Many of the nation's fifty-nine dental schools offer graduate programs in dental public health to provide dentists with postdoctoral education and field experience in preparation for work in this specialty area.

The program in dental public health at the University of Michigan is exemplary of the admission prerequisites and program of study required for preparation in this field. Elmer Green, who received his Master of Public Health degree (M.P.H.) from the University of Michigan in August 1972, described the program at the institution as follows:

> The residency program in dental public health includes selected formal academic courses and supervised practical experience tailored to the individual resident in research, administration, teaching, and epidemiology. The program is designed to increase the resident's competence in (a) planning, conducting, and evaluating dental public health programs; (b) serving as an effective member of the public health team; and (c) making contributions to the knowledge and advancement of the dental profession as it serves the public. The dental public health residency program also helps to meet requirements for application for examination by the American Board of Dental Public Health.
>
> Educational opportunities are available to residents in disciplines closely related to dental public health, such as biostatistics, epidemiology, health education, medical care, and behavioral sciences, as well as in specific advanced dental specialty fields.

Admission Requirements

Applicants for residency in dental public health must fulfill the following admission requirements:

1. to have received the Doctor of Dental Surgery (D.D.S.) degree or its equivalent from an accredited dental school;

2. to have graduated at least in the upper half (preferably the upper third) of the dental school class;

3. to have maintained a superior grade-point average

throughout the undergraduate and dental school programs;

4. to be licensed to practice in at least one state or territory of the United States (or equivalent certification for foreign students);

5. to complete the residency program to obtain certification by the American Board of Dental Public Health and to pursue a full-time career in dental public health practice and/or teaching;

6. to have stated objectives, in seeking residency, in harmony with this program.

Program of Study

The basic curriculum includes both course work in the several schools of the university and field experience in an approved or accredited institution or agency related to the needs and interests of the resident. The length of the program (from one-to-two years) is determined by these factors. Course work and practical experience are planned for each resident to build upon his particular background and objectives. Advanced training is provided until the objectives of both the programs and the resident are met and the resident is properly prepared to contribute to the field of dental public health. Upon completion of the study program, residents are expected to fill positions in official public health agencies or in educational institutions as administrators, teachers, or researchers.

Applicants also have the opportunity to work in programs which are designed to meet both the qualifications for the residency and for the M.P.H. degree. In addition, they may work in a combined program in dental public health and those for an advance degree offered by cooperating departments of the School of Public Health (if residents qualify and are admitted by the School to its degree program); e.g., the Doctor of Public Health (D.P.H.) degree through the Department of Epidemiology of the School of Public Health, or the Doctor of Philosophy (Ph.D.) degree or D.P.H. through the Department of Community Health Services.

Stipends are available to U.S. citizens or foreign nationals admitted to the United States for permanent residence at the following levels:

For first-year residents
with no postdoctoral training $6,000
with one year postdoctoral training   6,500
with two or more years postdoctoral
training.   7,000

In addition to the basic stipend, allowance is made in the amount of $500 per calendar year per dependent. Tuition is also provided.

Endodontics

Edodontics, the youngest specialty area, is that branch of dentistry concerned with the etiology, prevention, diagnosis, and treatment of diseases and injuries affecting the pulp and periapical tissues. The American Association of Endodontists (AAE) was founded in 1943.

There are several specialists (board eligible) and diplomates (certified by examination) among blacks:

Robert L. Ellison,* Detroit, Michigan
Raymond A. Hayes,* Ann Arbor, Michigan
David D. Parnell,* Columbus, Ohio
Daniel J. Whitner, Atlanta, Georgia
Bernard Whitsett,* Washington, D.C.
William J. Walker, Sr.*, Chicago, Illinois
William J. Walker, Jr., Framingham, Massachusetts
Herman F. Stamps,* Washington, D.C.
Jefferson J. Jones,* Cleveland, Ohio
Parker Wortham, Detroit, Michigan
John Mattox, Baltimore, Maryland
Matson Nelson, Nashville, Tennesee

------

*Board certified diplomates

Oral Pathology

The oral pathologist, concerned with the diagnosis of unusual diseases of the mouth, is not as well known to the public as some of the other specialists but is indispensible to the profession. Few blacks practice in this field, but inroads have been made. In 1957 Theodore E. Bolden became the first Meharry graduate to receive a Ph.D. degree in pathology from the University of Illinois. In that same year, Dr. Bolden became the first black appointed to the faculty of Seton Hall College of Medicine and Dentistry as assistant professor of oral pathology. In 1958 Daniel A. Collins became a diplomate of the American Board of Oral Pathology, the first black to have passed this Board.

Oral Surgery

Oral surgery includes the diagnosis and surgical treatment of injuries, diseases, and malformations of the jaws, and may range from the extraction of a tooth to the treatment of cysts, tumors, infections, and lesions of the mouth and jaws. More complex problems include jaw and facial injuries, repair of birth deformities of the lips and palate, and the surgical contouring of the mouth for better denture foundation.

To qualify as an oral surgeon, students must spend approximately eight years in college and dental school and be qualified as a general practitioner after which they must spend at least three more years in internship and residency programs in approved hospitals and universities.

Oral surgery often requires the use of hospital facilities, so a specialist in oral surgery is a member of the hospital staff. Most major hospitals have oral surgery services, thus an oral surgeon is prepared to provide for health care at the hospital as well as in his office.

In the past the black dentist seeking entrance to graduate oral surgery programs faced stiff racial barriers, but these barriers have lessened in recent years. A survey taken by C. Bassett Brown in 1969 of 157 approved graduate training programs (with a total of 284 openings each year) showed 64 blacks in 20 training programs completed one or more years of study (see Appendix I). Thirty programs never had a black apply, and 107 failed to respond to the survey. (All replies indicated that blacks would be considered with other applicants on an equal basis.) In 1969 there were 4,650 applicants for 481 positions, an indication of the severity of the competition.

After much debate and delay, the American Society of Oral Surgery (2,262 members) accepted Noah Calhoun as its first black member in 1961. There are now 14 black members, including Thomas Pinson, appointed an examiner for the society in 1969.

Founded in 1946, the American Board of Oral Surgery listed John Turner (1947) and Roscoe Lee (1948), both professors of oral surgery at Howard University, among its first 1,055 members. Samuel O. Banks of the department of oral surgery of Meharry School of Dentistry was accepted in 1951. There are 22 black oral surgeons practicing in the United States, but only 9 have successfully passed this board. (Dr. Calhoun has been appointed three times to the advisory committee, 1968-70.) A breakdown of these statistics shows that two are in hospital or Veteran's Administration service, one is in the U.S. Army and one was formerly in the Army: Lieutenant Colonel Harold W. Hargis, Chief Oral Surgeon and director of oral surgery training at William Beaumont General Hospital, El Paso, Texas. One is a full-time anesthetist. Four are part-time instructors, four head departments of oral surgery: J.B. Singleton (Meharry), James Stanback (Howard), Frank M. Lapeyrolerie (New Hersey College of Medicine and Dentistry), and Arthur Williams (Harlem Hospital). Thomas Pinson is associate dean at Howard University College of Dentistry; eight oral surgeons are in private practice. It also should be noted that at least twenty dentists with one year of oral surgery training are in general practice.

Oral surgery is a very rewarding specialty, for dental problems often require astute diagnosis and intricate surgical procedures. Oral surgeons are numbered among those earning the highest median income of all the dental specialties—$36,000 per year.

There is a critical demand for oral surgeons throughout the United States and a specific need for blacks to close the gap between the availability of their services and the needs of their people. Aid to students is available through the American Fund for Dental Health, a subsidiary of the ADA.

Orthodontics

Orthodontics is an area of dentistry concerned with the growth, guidance, correction, and maintenance of the dento-facial complex, with special emphasis on developmental disturbances and those conditions that cause or require movement of teeth. The practice of orthodontics includes the diagnosis, prevention, interception, and treatment of all forms of malocclusion (faulty closure of teeth) and the associated alteration in their supporting structures. It also includes the design, application, and control of functional corrective appliances and the guidance of the developing dentition to attain optimum occlusal relations in physiologic and esthetic harmony with other facial and cranial structures.

Orthodontics may be divided into three areas—preventive, interceptive, and corrective. The general practitioner is usually involved with preventive, interceptive, and limited corrective dentistry, but the orthodontist practices in all three areas.

Orthodontic Specialty Practice

Prevention of malocclusion is the primary responsibility of the orthodontist. Orthodontists welcome assistance from the general practitioner and other specialists in preventive dentistry, such as space maintenance, tooth preservation, and habit correction. However, all corrective procedures involving tooth movement and requiring either functional or mechanical treatment have been primarily orthodontics throughout the history of the specialty. The principal responsibility of the orthodontist is the supervision of the growth and development of the dentition and its associated facial structures, from birth through dental maturity.

In treating malocclusions, orthodontists seek to establish normal function and anatomical relations of the teeth and all of their supporting structures. This means that comprehensive training in the traditional areas of orthodontic practice is essential if the dentist or the orthodontist is to be fully competent to diagnose, design, and adjust the proper corrective appliance. He must continuously reevaluate the therapeutic procedures during the course of treatment and the subsequent period of retention.

TABLE 2
BLACK ORTHODONTISTS*

Name	Location
T. L. Alexander	Birmingham, Alabama
William J. Alexander	Washington, D.C.
Leonard Altemus	Washington, D.C.
Ernest W. Anderson	Washington, D.C.
James M. Bailey, Jr.	Takoma Park, Maryland
Richard Bean	Washington, D.C.
William Benjamin, Jr.	Washington, D.C.
William J. Bryant	Boston, Massachusetts
Ralph A. Callender	Los Angeles, California
Herbert M. Campbell	Dayton, Ohio
Ruth D. Carter	Los Angeles, California
Wendell Cotton	Lompoc, California
Gwendolyn F. Dunn	Baltimore, Maryland
John Egan	Detroit, Michigan
Clarence C. Evans	Washington, D.C.
Roscoe C. Foster	Chicago, Illinois
LaForrest Garner	Indianapolis, Indiana
Larry J. Green	Buffalo, New York
Elisha J. Greenfield	Chicago, Illinois
Frank Harris	Detroit, Michigan
Charles Hawkins	Middletown, Ohio
Charles F. Johnson	Atlanta, Georgia
Glenwood Jordan	Houston, Texas
Harry M. McLinn	New York, New York
Timothy C. Meyers	Atlanta, Georgia
Byron L. Mitchell	Miami, Florida
Richard Morgan	Boston, Massachusetts

BLACK ORTHODONTISTS (continued)

Name	Location
Clarence Red	Chicago, Illinois
Earl W. Renfroe	Chicago, Illinois
Elisha R. Richardson	Nashville, Tennessee
Donald Russell	West Indies
Richard Simms	Los Angeles, California
Randolph W. Sturrup	Houston, Texas
Roland Thomas	Chicago, Illinois
Duncan J. Thorne	New York, New York
Mitchell N. Toney	Cleveland, Ohio
Alphonso Trottman	St. Louis, Missouri
Elgin E. Wells	Houston, Texas
Claude R. Williams	Dallas, Texas
Harvey J. Williams	Pacoima, California

Source: Elisha R. Richardson, chairman, Department of Orthodontics, Meharry Medical College School of Dentistry, Nashville, Tennessee.

*The orthodontists listed above have met the minimum standards of at least eighteen months of postdoctoral study in orthodontics on a full-time basis.

Orthodontics for the General Dentist

The general practitioner is frequently involved in preventive, interceptive, and limited corrective orthodontics. Preventive orthodontics refer to the elimination of factors that may lead to malocclusion in an otherwise normally developing dentition. Interceptive orthodontics refers to the correction of conditions that are not considered to be major problems. Limited corrective orthodontics involves minor tooth movement procedures in patients who have basically normal occlusions. The general dentist guides the occlusion and makes minor modifications contributing to the normal development of the dental arches.

Admissions Requirements and Program of Study

Orthodontics is a specialty that prides itself on excellence and accepts only top-quality candidates as graduate students. Currently, a student should be in the upper tenth of his or her class to be assured of getting into the program. However, those in the upper half of the class also have a reasonable chance of being admitted. In essence, if students consider careers in orthodontics, they must start early to acquire good study habits and the academic background necessary to succesfully pursue the discipline and its related basic sciences in dental college.

In 1971 there were forty-nine schools in the U.S. offering formal orthodontic training or educational programs, and three in Canada.[1] There were also two programs of residency. The minimum course is eighteen months; the average course is twenty-four months.

Blacks in the Field

The first black to complete training in orthodontics was Earl W. Renfroe, a 1941 graduate of the University of Illinois. He was also the first black to be certified by the American Board of Orthodontics (ABO).

At the present time, three blacks chair postgraduate or graduate orthodontic departments: Earl W. Renfroe (University of Illinois), Richard Beane (Howard University), and LaForrest D. Garner (Indiana University). The undergraduate department of Meharry Medical College is chaired by Elisha R. Richardson.

Among the more than 6,500 orthodontists in the United States, there are only approximately 30 blacks, seven of which are certified by the ABO: Leonard Altemus, LaForrest D. Garner, Harry McLinn, Matthew Mitchell, Earl W. Renfroe, Elisha R. Richardson, and Richard Simms. (Dr. Mitchell is deceased.)

In addition to private practice, black orthodontists are needed in teaching, research, and other institutional activities, especially in cities with a large black population.

Pedodontics

Pedodontics involves treatment of all oral health conditions in children, except those irregularities requiring major orthodontic treatment or surgery.

The prevention of disease and good dental care in early

childhood are matters of special concern for the black dentists and reasons for the large number of blacks currently entering this specialty. In 1961 A. M. Pratt of Chicago, a diplomate of the Illinois Board of Pedodontics, was the first black certified as a pedodontist. Dr. Pratt holds the patent of the simplex matrix retainer (a dental instrument) and is a contributor to *Health For All,* currently used as a text in the Chicago public school system. Dr. Pratt is also author of *Your Children, Their Teeth and Their Health.* [2]

Gary H. Radford, Jr., a pedodontist in Houston, Texas, noted that there were approximately eight black students in pedodontic residency programs who would complete postgraduate training during the 1975-76 academic year.

An assistant professor of pedodontics at Louisiana State University School of Dentistry in New Orleans, Clifton O. Dummett, Jr., became the first black member of that faculty in May 1975. He also serves as coordinator for pedodontic extra-mural activity and departmental research and is chief of pedodontics at Charity Hospital in that city.

Periodontics

During the 1950s and 1960s, more blacks entered the field of periodontics than ever before. In 1959 the U.S. Public Health Service awarded an $80,000 grant to G. W. Wade of Howard University for a five-year study of the role of saliva in healing mouth wounds. In 1962, Marion George Ford, Jr., of Houston, Texas, was awarded a Fulbright fellowship to study periodontology at the University of Bonn, Germany, the first black in that area of study to receive a Fulbright and the first dentist of either race to be so honored in Texas.

Other awards and achievements by blacks in the field were: presentation by the American Public Health Association of its forty-year membership certificate to Roscoe C. Brown of Washington, D.C. (1959), publication in *Journal of the Tennessee State Dental Association* (January 1960) of an important study by Eugenia L. Mobley (D.D.S.) and Martha Pointer (M.A.), "Dental Caries and Periodontal Conditions among Negro Children in Tennessee."

Another important study was presented in March 1963 at a meeting of the International Association of Dental Research by Andrew Z. Keller, a Harvard dental graduate with a M.P.H. degree from Johns Hopkins University in epidemiology and a member of the Public Health Research Institute of New York. In this study, "The Epidemiology of Lip, Oral, and Pharyngeal Cancers and the Associations with Selected Systemic Diseases," Dr. Keller observed that men who develop cancer in the floor of the mouth have a marked tendency to suffer from cirrhosis of the liver. The study also showed that lip cancer is extremely rare in blacks but occurs with unusual frequency among white males, especially inhabitants of the South and West. He also found that upper lip cancer occurs with less frequency than lower lip cancer, and at an earlier age.

Prosthodontics

Almost all dentists practice some prosthodontics—the design and construction of dental appliances and substitutes for natural teeth. However, the 1973 statistics from the ADA Bureau of Economics, Research, and Statistics show that only 702 out of 102,978 dentists in the United States practice this specialty exclusively.

The percentage of black dentists engaged in this specialty is also small, although several black dentists pioneered in this area and demonstrated remarkable knowledge and skill in lectures, clinics, and postgraduate courses so that their colleagues were inspired to follow in their footsteps.

Some pioneers in this field were: Robert F. Sanford, Professor of prosthetic dentistry, Meharry Medical College School of Dentistry; William H. Allen, dean of the Meharry School; Percy Fitzgerald, professor of prosthodontics, Howard University; R. M. Reddick, Columbus, Georgia; D. H. Turpin, Meharry; I. D. Moore, Chicago, Illinois; E. W. Taggert, Birmingham, Alabama; and Adolphous Walton, Howard University.

In 1965 the first black to become a diplomate of the American Board of Prosthodontics was James T. Jackson, associate dean for clinical affairs and visiting professor of prosthodontics, Howard University College of Dentistry. Dr. Jackson, who is also associate professor of prosthodontics at Georgetown University, has lectured on prosthodontics at many other universities in this country and abroad.

Chapter V

Women in Dentistry

Approximately 1,100 women in the United States were engaged in the private practice of dentistry in 1976, comprising 1.2 percent of the total profession. However, less than 1 percent of these women are black. In many European countries, women dentists considerably outnumber males in the profession; for example, in Russia 70 percent of all dentists are women. Finland has an even greater number, 80 percent; Greece and Denmark, 40-50 percent; and France, Germany, Norway, and Sweden, 35 percent each. These figures reveal that the dental profession is definitely not exclusively a male province.

Great strides are being taken in America to remove the stereotype of the male dentist, but of the 16,000 students enrolled in dental schools in 1969, only 174 were women. In addition, in the same years, fewer than 100 women were numbered among the 10,000 applicants for dental school, according to the ADA's Council on Dental Education. Yet statistics reveal that 41.6 percent of the women over sixteen years of age are in the U.S. labor force; five percent of practicing lawyers and eight percent of practicing physicians are women.

Although the percentage of women studying dentistry has increased 489 percent in the past five years, according to an ADA report the number of women is still fewer than the number of men entering the profession. Perhaps this results from the fact that few women have a clear idea of the scope and objectives of modern dentistry. The average person thinks of dentistry in terms of the mechanical phases only. One hundred years ago this may have been the case, but today dentistry is an important health service. Emphasis has shifted from restoration to prevention; the modern dentist diagnoses, prescribes and treats oral health conditions.

The newer concept of dental disease and its relation to general bodily and mental health has greatly affected the theory and practice of dentistry. It has made the dentist an important member of a health team, consisting of the physician, the dentist, the nurse, the dental hygienist, and various technical assistants, all of whom work in close cooperation to maintain, improve, and restore health.

Modern dentistry is not practiced by the application of brute force. The strength required is easily within the range of a normal, healthy female. The size and dexterity of a woman's

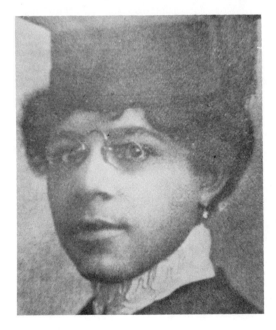

Dr. Ollie L. Bryan was the first woman to graduate from Meharry Medical College and the first black woman to practice dentistry in the South in the early 1900s.

hands and fingers are anatomical advantages which foster mastery of motor skills in the comparatively small working area of the human mouth.

Despite the great advances in dental practice, many questions remain unanswered, and there is still a great need for investigation and discovery. Unlimited horizons are open to the young woman with imagination and energy. Any female who can master the prerequisite sciences on an equal basis with her male counterpart will find no difficulty in acquiring the basic knowledge for dental practice. A mature student who succeeds in biology or chemistry will have no serious difficulty in learning preclinical subjects. Once these are mastered, the acquisition and integration of clinical knowledge and experience is much easier.

No woman should assume that riches are to be had for the asking in the profession, but the dentist makes an above-average income. It is difficult to predict how well any individual will succeed, but nearly two-thirds of the nation's dentists earn net incomes of more than $20,000 per year; one quarter, a net income of more than $30,000; and some specialists, more than $40,000.

Early Women Dentists

The first woman to enter the profession in the United States was Emeline Roberts Jones of Connecticut. At the age of seventeen, she married a dentist and became his assistant. After his death in 1864, she developed a growing practice of her own and became a member of the Women's Advisory Council at the World's Columbian Dental Congress of 1893.

Lucy Hobbs of Iowa was admitted to Ohio Dental College as early as 1866, although by the time of her graduation in 1870, there were twenty-four women practicing dentistry in the United States. It is believed, however, that Dr. Hobbs was the only woman to receive formal training and to graduate from a dental college of that time. (In 1880, there were 611 women dentists; in 1890, 337. By 1920 women constituted 3 percent of the total practicing dentistry.)

Dr. Ida Gray Nelson Rollins was the first black woman to receive a dental degree in the United States. Born between 1865 and 1867 in Tennessee, Ida Gray grew up and attended public schools in Cincinnati, Ohio, graduating from high school in 1887. She enrolled in the University of Michigan Dental School in 1887 and received the degree of D.D.S. in 1890. From 1890 to 1895, Dr. Ida Gray practiced dentistry in Cincinnati, Ohio. She married James S. Nelson in 1895 and they moved to Chicago where she lived the rest of her life.

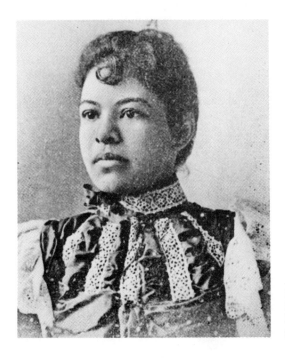

Dr. Ida Gray Nelson Rollins was the first black female dentist to hold a degree.

As Dr. Ida Gray Nelson, she was known to be active in several women's organizations in Chicago and was frequently cited as an example of what woman could become. Her first husband, James Sanford Nelson, was an accountant and attorney and also served as an officer in the Eighth Illinois National Guard unit. He saw active duty in both the Spanish-American-Cuban and First World Wars. He died March 11, 1926. In 1929, Ida Gray Nelson married William A. Rollins and she was known thereafter as Dr. Ida N. Rollins. She remained married to Mr. Rollins until his death on June 20, 1944.

It appears that Dr. Ida N. Rollins was still known as a practicing dentist in the mid-1930's. She died on May 3, 1953. Dr. Rollins was apparently proud of her distinction as witnessed by the inscription on her gravestone: "Dr. Ida Gray Nelson Rollins, 1st Negro Woman Dentist in America."

TABLE 3
NEGRO WOMEN DENTISTS

Name	Location	Year of Graduation
Ida Gray Nelson	Illinois	1895
Mary Imogene Williams	District of Columbia	1896
Alva C. Garrot	(Deceased)	1899
A. Marie Waring	New York	1900
Ollie L. Bryan	Texas	1900(?)
Gertrude Curtis	New York	1909
Mary H. Shetton	Texas	1910(?)
Edna Corrine Robinson	New York	1916
Alice Watkins Garrott	California	1917
Mary Jane Watkins	New York	1917
Vada Jetmore Sommerville	California	1918
Addie Williams	New York	1921
Clarice B. Allen	Texas	1924
Julia Arnette Freeman	(Deceased)	1924
Zelma Holmes	Kentucky	1926
Anna C. Johnson	New York	1927
Marie Hackley	Michigan	1928
Racheal Ellis	New York	1928
Hazel M. Moore	Arkansas	1930
Stephanie Davis	New York	1932
Olive Lee Burks Hine	New York	1933
Ferris Warren	New York	1935
Donzleigh J. Cann	Bermuda	1936
Mildred Florine Edwards	Tennessee	1941
Kathryn White	Tennessee	1943
Sara Archie Lee	Accra, Ghana, W.A.	1945

NEGRO WOMEN DENTISTS (continued)

Name	Location	Year of Graduation
Dorothy M. Reed	New York	1945
Helen M. Guenever Smith	California	1946
Eugenia Mobley McGinnis	Tennesse	1946
Vivian Dowell	Oklahoma	1947
Mavis N. Jones	Mississippi	1948
Electra D. Green	Ohio	1948
Ruth Durley Carter	California	1948
Grace E. Byrd	(Deceased)	1948
Evangeline Upshur Freeman	Arkansas	1949
Virginia Gladding Jones		1950
Etta G. Gopaul		1951
Violet M. London	New York	1951
Clifton Jones		1951
Rosey P. Sheik		1951
Bertha M. Martin	District of Columbia	1951
Ellen Q. Smith	Tennessee	1951
Patricia Louise Shook	California	1951
Rosalie R. Miller	Washington	1951
Nancy C. Gannaway	North Carolina	1954
Kathleen J. Gordon Tomlinson		1954
Dorotha E. Hill (Lemeh)	Massachusetts	1954
Gertrude H. Garnes Paxton	California	1956
Lee Toh Tan Hcsannah		1956
Vera Strong Anderson	Ohio	1957
Lyvonne Mackel Washington	Indiana	1957
Frances C. Lee Young	District of Columbia	1958
Florence McNeill	District of Columbia	1958
Gloria J. Robinson		1958
Jacqueline D. Guinn	Ohio	1958
Jeanne C. Sinkford	District of Columbia	1958
Betty Cobb Jones	Maryland	1959
Mary N. Kagwa	Kampala, Uganda, E. Africa	1960
Louise W. Watson		1960
Mabel W. Robinson	New Jersey	1960
Jacqueline D. Steward	District of Columbia	1961
Susie Chapman	Georgia	1961
Nona Baird	Illinois	1962
Juliann S. Bluitt	Illinois	1962
Diane Harris	Virginia	1962
Bobbie J. Raleigh	District of Columbia	1962

NEGRO WOMEN DENTISTS (continued)

Name	Location	Year of Graduation
Joyce A. Reese Peagler	District of Columbia	1963
Shirley A. Jordan Bailey	New York	1964
Mariam Ibrahim Khatri	Indiana	1965
Millicent Henry	Indiana	1965
Grace E. Robinson	Maryland	1965
Thermutel A. Lobban	District of Columbia	1966
Ann L. Bryan	District of Columbia	1967
Helen Burrell	New Jersey	1969
Ethell Jackson	District of Columbia	1969
Tamara Ewell Jackson	Pennsylvania	1969
Patricia Niles	District of Columbia	1970
Cecile Ganpatzingh	Massachusetts	1968
Maysa Mesa	New Jersey	1972
Marbara Sias	Mississippi	1973
Ruth Anderson	Pennsylvania	1973
Evelyn Wiley	Oklahoma	1973
Sandra Berry	Tennessee	1973
Melba Wilson	Texas	1973
Linda Lott	Texas	1973
Muthoni Gitata	Kenya	1973
Shirley Murphy	Massachusetts	1975

Source: Clifton O. Dummett, *Growth and Development of the Negro in Dentistry in the United States* (Chicago: The Stanek Press, 1952). Additional names were supplied by Drs. Jeanne C. Sinkford, Eugenia Mobley, Mary Jane Watkins, Juliann S. Bluitt, and Melba Wilson.

Chapter VI

Dental Auxiliaries

The Dental Hygienist

Traditionally, the hygienist's role as a practicing member of the dental team consists of helping to maintain healthy mouths, teeth, and gums, and preventing dental disorders. The hygienist is also trained to perform two primary functions in the prevention and treatment of disease: scaling and polishing the natural and restored surfaces of the teeth, applying caries retardment agents, and performing diagnostic, clinical and laboratory tests. In addition, the hygienist instructs patients about the importance of maintaining sound teeth, including diet as a means of insuring dental health and preventing caries. He or she also executes basic procedures to control dental disease caused by plaque.

A dental hygienist must graduate from a high school offering college preparatory courses, with an above-average academic record. While requirements vary, most hygiene programs require strong academic background in mathematics and the sciences, including biology and chemistry. Beyond high school, many students enroll in two- or three-year college programs which award certificates or associate degrees. Others choose to enroll in four-year baccalaureate programs. In addition, those desiring further study to assure additional opportunities for advancement must complete the master's degree.

Graduates of two- or three-year certificate or associate degree programs are generally limited to dental office practice and some public health positions, although they may later elect to continue to the baccalaureate or master's degree. Hygienists with bachelor's degrees may enter private practice and, with office experience, are eligible for dental hygiene teaching or administrative public health positions. The master's degree prepares the dental hygienist for advanced positions in teaching, administration, and public health. After graduation, dental hygienists earn an above-average salary, and as a career, the field offers versatility in its various procedures and multiple opportunities.

The relative absence of blacks and other minority groups from the profession can probably be attributed to sociological and economic factors, as well as to the general lack of awareness of the potential of this relatively new profession, and the inadequate career guidance and counseling. (Nine out of ten of today's minority hygienists are graduates of Howard or Meharry dental schools, each of which has had an accredited hygiene program since 1951.)

The relatively small ratio of dentists (1-to-17) who employ hygienists indicates that increased efforts are needed to provide information about dental hygiene as a career choice. The recent growth of the number of programs (from 30 to 102) and the increased enrollment (2,500 to 6,000) during the past decade, indicates the increasing popularity of the profession. Although statistics are not available on the percentage of this number who are minority students, it is certain that the group is quite small.

Recent testimony before the Senate Subcommittee on Health stated that the dental profession has long recognized the essential role played by the dental auxiliaries, but there have never been, nor are there now, adequate numbers to fill the need for 5,500 additional hygienists required annually. Our present educational system must prepare more students to meet the future manpower needs of the profession. Statistics and trends indicate that the demand will be great for these services and for the utilization of dental auxiliaries. Whether the role of the hygienist as it is known today remains the same and whether, in fact, this auxiliary retains its current title, the hygienist will continue to play an important and vital role in the profession as a stalwart in providing preventive treatment services.

Furthermore, if the United States is to fulfill the responsibility of making health care (of which dental care is certainly an important part) a basic right of all citizens, it is logical to assume that there must be increased and more effective emphasis on all areas of preventive medicine and hygiene.

The Dental Assistant

In 1885, a New Orleans dentist employed a young woman to replace a black man in his office—a startling innovation of that time. This early experiment gradually led to the conclusion that women had the proper amount of native intelligence as well as other talents of great assistance to any dentist who had the temerity to employ them. Still, the employment of women in dental offices was not generally accepted for some time. Finally, windows of dental offices exhibited placards stating "Lady in Attendance," thus making it respectable for a woman to go to a dental office unaccompanied. But the employment of women continued to be vigorously debated among dentists for a number of years. Today, dental assistants are almost exclusively women, although men, of course, are encouraged to join the practice.

The first organization of dental assistants, founded in 1921 in New York City by Juliette A. Southard, was called the Education and Efficiency Society. In 1924, Mrs. Southard also founded the American Dental Assistants Association (ADAA), which now offers a 104-hour study course in every district as preparation for the examination of the state certification committees. The National Dental Association of Negro Dental Assistants was organized in Cleveland, Ohio, August 3, 1964 during a NDA convention.

The real function of a dental assistant is service: readying patients for dental treatment, assisting the dentist at the chair, and preparing dental materials. The dental assistant also assumes secretarial duties, performs laboratory procedures, and handles appointments and financial arrangements. In fact, the efficient operation of a dental office depends on the capability of the dental assistant.

For many years, on-the-job training was the only means by which one could learn the trade, but today, the dental assistant is urged to continue his or her education through every possible means. Dental anatomy, radiology, ethics and jurisprudence, dental science, and many other courses must be taken to meet the requirements for certification. As a member of local, state, and national organizations, the dental assistant must take advantage of the many programs available to increase his or her interest, knowledge, skill, and understanding of various phases of the job.

A wide variety of employment choices are available: private dental practice, group dental practice, hospital dental service, government service, and dental assistance education. Alabama grants dental assistants the right to take the State Dental Board Examination to become licensed dental hygienists. For a while the state of Georgia did also. In 1948 Louise Rucker, working in the dental office of L. V. Reese, Sr., of Atlanta, took advantage of this opportunity and became the first black licensed dental hygienist in that state. However, Georgia no longer permits preceptorship training for dental hygienists, and in Alabama, this practice is now under attack by the Alabama Dental Hygienists' Association.

The Dental Technician

Dental laboratory technology is the art of constructing artificial or prosthetic dental restorations. The field can be divided into the following general areas: partial and complete dentures, crown and fixed bridgework, porcelain and acrylic restorations, and orthodontic appliances.

The dental technician has the same relationship to the dentist as the pharmacist has to the physician and the optician to the ophthalmologist. As a member of the dental health team, the technician's skills and knowledge are an invaluable aid to its success.

Dental technicians are employed in some 7,500 commercial dental laboratories in the United States, while approximately 2,500 work for dentists in private practice and 650 are employed by the federal government. In all, there are approximately 25,000 technicians in the United States, serving more than 110,000 dentists. In addition to the increasing national population and the number of older citizens who require extensive dental health care, there is the growing public awareness of the importance of preventive dentistry. An estimated 30,000,000 Americans expect to be covered by dental care insurance during the next ten years, hence it is easy to imagine the magnitude of the challenges and opportunities available to young people entering this field. Salaries range up to $21,000 per annum for master technologists in managerial positions, from $12,000 per annum for experienced licensed technicians.

Although a high school education is sufficient to pursue this career, a higher educational level is desirable. In addition, a candidate should have special skills, such as a high degree of manual dexterity, good color perception, and a preference for detailed work. (Applicants whose avocations are painting, ceramics, sculpture, and related fields generally become proficient dental technicians.)

Dental laboratory training is offered at community colleges or dental schools with two-year courses, at private schools, and in on-the-job training programs in laboratories. Norman Dental Laboratories, Inc., New York City—the largest dental laboratory in the nation owned by blacks—offers a training program for disadvantaged youth funded by the U.S. Department of Labor. The National Association of Certified Dental Laboratories, of which Norman is a member, sponsors a nine-month training program in dental technology. Also, the United States Army, Navy, and Air Force have training programs in dental laboratory technology.

Many organizations and corporations have made grants and

scholarships available to qualified candidates through The Fund for Dental Health. In addition, a number of scholarships are available at schools accredited by the ADA.

It has become apparent that the boom in population and the demands for dental treatment are increasing faster than the number of new dentists entering the practice. The profession must rely more and more upon other members of the dental health team: the technician, the hygienist, and the assistant. It is almost mandatory today that practicing dentists—with the objective of spending more time at the chair—add dental technicians to their staffs and utilize more fully the services of commercial laboratories.

Chapter VII

The Black Dentist and

the Military

Prior to 1918 few black dentists were commissioned to serve as officers in the Armed Forces. Edward L. Grant, a 1913 graduate of Meharry College of Dentistry and licensed practitioner in the St. Louis, Missouri area, was drafted into the army as a private and discharged as a private. Records do not reveal any blacks serving on active duty as commissioned officers between World War I and World War II. It was not until 1942 that a concentrated effort was made to train or recruit black dental officers.

Even during World War II the Army was segregated, and the majority of medical officers serving in black units were white, including those who served in the two largest black divisions, the 92nd and 93rd Infantry. In June 1940, when mobilization began, the War Department recorded only eight black dentists eligible for active duty, and the four tactical units with black troops could assign only five dental officers. Consequently, large numbers of black dentists began seeking appointments in the Reserves as commissioned officers. However, they too were rejected and forced to serve as infantrymen or in positions outside of their specialties.

Army Specialty Training Program

The advent of the Army Specialty Training Program (ASTP)

in the early 1940s began to correct some of the military's discriminatory practices and provided an avenue by which many black men could enter the dental profession. This government-sponsored program was put into effect at many dental schools, including Howard and Meharry. During this program, black graduates were admitted to dental colleges for an accelerated three-year program and commissioned to serve in the Army as dental officers after graduation. This program made new career opportunities financially possible for many black dentists.

At the end of World War II, more than ninety black dentists had served as professionals in the Army, and many had been placed in hospitals or dispensaries outside of black units. The average rank held by black dentists at the end of the war was captain, although at this time there were also three majors and one lieutenant colonel.

Air Force and Navy

In 1947 members of the Army Medical Corps were given the choice of remaining in the Army or joining the Medical Corps of the new U.S. Air Force. Many dentists elected to become officers in the Air Force. The Armed Forces had been totally integrated by order of the late President Harry S. Truman, but it is not known whether a black dentist was in the first group of Air Force doctors. When Virdumarus Nickols entered the Air Force after several years of experience as an Army enlisted man, he was the oldest known living black military dentist. The first black woman dentist to be commissioned in the U.S. Air Force was Lt. Raya Rachlin, a 1952 graduate of Howard University College of Dentistry.

In the early 1950s the United States became involved in the Korean War. To meet the quota of professional dentists needed, the so-called "Doctor Draft" was enacted. Many blacks were drafted into the Army, but some volunteered for service in the Navy to avoid the draft. It was during this time that the Navy commissioned its first black dental officer, Lt. Thomas L. James, a 1951 graduate of Meharry. Lt. (j.g.) Thomas Watkins, Jr., was the first black dentist commissioned in the U.S. Naval Reserve Dental Corps. Lt. Watkins was an honor graduate in dentistry of the Class of 1944 at the University of Pennsylvania.

Today, black dentists serve in every branch of military service, in every specialty. The greatest number of doctors enter the military with the rank of captain, serve their two year obligation, and return to civilian life. Presently, more than one percent of the dentists in the military are black; the highest rank is colonel. Although a black dentist has never been promoted to general rank in any branch of the military, there have been many high-ranking dental specialists and several consultants to the Dental Surgeon. Col. Coleman Tuckson, U.S. Air Force Reserve (Washington, D.C.), has served as Dental Radiologist and Consultant to the Air Force Dental Surgeon.

Though the United States military has had great impact on blacks in dentistry, it has denied full and complete access to the upper echelon of rank and privilege.

Chapter VIII

Black Dentists and

the Community

Black health professionals are noted for their community involvement and leadership in all phases of public life. The dentist is no exception. For as long as the practice of dentistry has had professional status, blacks have been involved in oral health concerns of their own communities and the nation as a whole.

John S. Rock, a native of Salem, New Jersey—physician, dentist, lawyer, and one of the best-educated blacks of the pre-Civil War period—was well known for his views on anti-slavery issues and equal rights. He opposed all proposals to settle black Americans abroad, and in 1862, addressed members of the Massachusetts Anti-Slavery Society against various colonizing proposals. Even though the nation had discriminated against blacks for nearly two-and-a-half centuries and now wished them to leave, Dr. Rock encouraged his audience to stay in America, "to pay-off the old score, and have a reconstruction of things."[1]

Before the turn of the century, J.R. Porter, while enjoying an excellent dental practice in Birmingham, Alabama, sought closer ties with the community. He founded the Penny Savings Bank of Birmingham and became the first secretary of its Board of Directors. Dr. Porter graduated in 1886 with an A.B. degree from Atlanta University, and after one year, entered the dental department of Walden University (at that time, Central Tennessee College). He received the degree of D.D.S. in 1889. The following year, he became a professor of operative dentistry at his alma mater. Porter was an indispensable leader in the public and religious life of the community. He was very much concerned with the future of young blacks and served as an officer in the local Y.M.C.A. Later, Dr. Porter moved to Atlanta, Georgia, where he built another outstanding dental practice and continued his community activities.

One of Porter's contemporaries, D. Watson Onley, was a prime example of adaptability and courage. In 1885, before entering dental school, he had been an architect and builder in Jacksonville, Florida. After three years of prosperous business, he opened the first steam saw and planing mill owned and operated entirely by blacks. The plant, which manufactured building lumber, grew rapidly, increased its facilities, and prospered until it was set afire by an arsonist.

At that time the State Normal and Industrial College needed a practical and efficient man to take charge of its technical department and solicited Onley's services. He accepted a position to teach all branches of architectural and mechanical drawing, manual training, operation of woodworking machinery, and the steam engine.

After some time Onley became dissatisfied with this new endeavor and entered the field of dentistry. After three years of hard study, struggle, and sacrifice, in addition to the responsibilities of a growing family, Onley completed his dental studies at Howard University and thereafter opened a practice in Washington, D.C.

Another black dentist, Haley Bell of Detroit, Michigan, was probably the first black to open an office in the predominantly Polish community of Hamtramck, Michigan. He began his practice in 1923, one year after graduation from Meharry Medical College. At that time, many blacks were leaving the South to find jobs in Detroit's auto factories, and Bell, with his wife, joined the exodus.

While waiting to take the Michigan State Dental examination, Bell worked at various unrelated jobs, but soon found a position in the office of a white dentist. After six months, he opened his own office in Hamtramck. There he developed a practice that was 97 percent white. It remained that way from its inception January 1924 until Bell's retirement in 1960.

Dr. Bell was always concerned about community problems and created many jobs for young blacks. After World War II he opened a tool and die shop and two trade schools, the Midway Technical School in New York and the Motor City Trade School in Detroit. With the help of other leading citizens of Detroit, he also taught young men the cleaning and pressing business.

Other problems of blacks interested Bell, especially those involving adjustment to city life. He encouraged a minister to start a listener-supported radio program to educate blacks, and eventually, when the minister became tired of writing the scripts, Bell considered buying his own station.

Although many friends tried to discourage Bell, a black who owned a small amount of stock in a southern radio station assured Bell that blacks would support a black-owned radio station. Subsequently, Bell began to investigate opening such a station in Detroit. Although the FCC had not granted any requests for new stations in the area for eleven years, in 1955 Bell bypassed Detroit and made a successful request for a station in Inkster, a western suburb.

Meanwhile, Bell's son-in-law, Wendell Cox—also a dentist—joined Bell in forming the Bell Broadcasting System. The station's call letters, WCHB, were taken from the initials of the two dentists.

Later, Bell Broadcasting Company opened SCHB-FM. These two radio stations answered the needs of blacks in providing fast communication, plus management that understood and sympathized with the black community. WCHB made free air time available to women's causes and church and fraternal organizations. In addition, it was the major outlet for the talent of young black artists who would never have been heard otherwise. WCHB also recognized the recording efforts of Berry Gordy, the owner of Motown Industries, and consistently played his company's records.

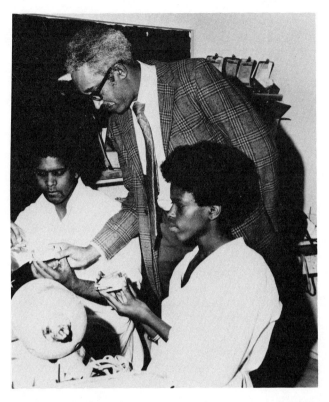

Norman D. Halliburton (second from right) inspects work of his technicians at his Norman Dental Laboratories, New York City.

Bell's sons-in-law, Drs. Wendell Cox and C. Robert Bass, both dentists, worked closely with him in establishing these stations as major forces in the black community; which employed more than fifty persons in 1976. Bell was also prominent in many other business and civic activities: the Victory Mutual Life Insurance Company. He was also a large contributor to the United Negro College Fund, the NAACP, and the United Foundation, and assisted many young people in educational pursuits before his death in January 1973.

In 1940 Lonnie E. Smith, a dentist of Houston, Texas, filed suit in a federal court on behalf of himself and other blacks whose basic civil right to vote had been denied. (At that time blacks could not participate in the Texas primary elections.) With the help of NAACP lawyers, Smith tenaciously fought this battle until a decision was rendered in his favor on April 4. Another prominant black in the political arena was Vernon E. Rice of Kansas City, Missouri, a 1963 graduate of Meharry Medical College School of Dentistry. As the Republican candidate for Congress in the Fifth District, Dr. Rice's key issues were education, busing, and welfare reform.

Across the nation, other black dentists were assuming leadership roles in politics. In Oklahoma City, the Oklahoma State Pardon and Parole Board elected its first black chairman in 1966. Dr. Robert B. Taylor, Jr., of Okmulgee was unanimously selected to head the clemency review committee. A trustee of the College of the Ozarks, Clarksville, Arkansas, Taylor is also a member of the Okmulgee Board of Education and director of the Chamber of Commerce, in their city, as well as a member of the Board of Directors of the Public Service Company of Oklahoma. In 1970 Taylor received the Thomas Jefferson Citizen's Award conferred annually on a member of the dental profession who has made significant contributions to civic and community affairs in Oklahoma.

In April, 1966, G. H. Radford, Sr., was elected to the Waco, Texas, city council and served three terms, one year as mayor *pro tem.* In Gainesville, Georgia, E. A. Cosby was elected chairman of the Housing Authority for a one year term in 1967. He also served on the City Planning Board for more than two years.

The first black to seek the governorship of the State of Alabama in 68 years was a dentist, John L. Chashin, Jr., of Huntsville, who founded the National Democratic Party of Alabama in 1968. He was Chairman of that party which served as a vehicle through which blacks could achieve representative government. In an interview in the Birmingham *Post Herald* on September 15, 1970, Cashin discussed his dual careers. "My profession has been dedicated to the relief of pain, and I have found that in wanting to serve and take care of the needs of people I have been more effective in the streets than in dentistry. I can remove one abscess in the dental chair, but I can remove a lot of abscesses of soul and mind in one fell swoop in politics."

"The cancer of racism," Cashin continued, "deliberately implanted, is the most effective political weapon in the South. If I can surgically remove this cancer, I will be very proud. . . ."

The Huntsville dentist has never sought office before, but had long been active in the Alabama civil rights movement and was a former state chairman of the NAACP. His chances for beating the incumbent, Governor George Wallace, were slim. Leading a ticket of over 170, Cashin felt that at least two-thirds of the black candidates who entered the race would be elected. Although Cashin himself was unsuccessful in winning the gubernatorial candidacy, his party voted a number of blacks into high offices in the state.

Another black dentist to run for governor in the Deep South was Reginald A. Hawkins of North Carolina. While Hawkins did not succeed in the 1968 election, he won one out of every five votes cast. (Hawkins again lost the race for governor in 1972.) His campaign provided an opportunity to raise critical questions about such issues as poverty and racism, which affected and continue to affect many of the citizens of North Carolina. Dr. Hawkins also questioned the inadequate political representation of many segments of the population. Hence one worthwhile result of his campaign was the formation of the North Carolina Committee for more Representative Political Participation. This group, headed by Hawkins, challenged the North Carolina Democratic Party in 1968 at the National Convention, demanding at least proportionate political representation of the blacks. One of the reforms now undertaken by the North Carolina Democratic Party and the National Democratic Party is precisely that of ensuring adequate representation, based upon race, age, and sex.

Another staunch fighter in the civil rights struggle at the local community level was Errold Duncan St. George Collymore, a resident of White Plains, New York. A native of Bridgetown,

Barbados, Collymore lived in White Plains for 46 years until his death in 1972. He organized the White Plains NAACP and founded the United Republican Club in that city, while waging a successful campaign against racial discrimination at Grasslands Hospital for the admission of black nurses and nursing students to that Westchester County facility. Collymore also broke racial barriers in the Ninth District Dental Society and the White Plains Dental Forum by successfully obtaining membership in both organizations. In addition, he was active in the Boy Scouts organization, the Parent-Teacher Association, and as a member of the Board of Directors of the Westchester Urban league for more than thirty years. For his outstanding services to the community, Dr. Collymore was presented the Leibman Brothers Good Neighbor Award in 1961. He also helped to integrate the religious life of White Plains by joining the Community Church (Unitarian), where he served as secretary of the Board of Trustees and director of the American Unitarian Association. He continued to be active in these community endeavors until his death in 1972.

Much more remains to be said about the thrust and influence of the black dentist in his community. James W. Holley, 3rd, president of the NDA summed it up very succinctly in his 1970 annual message to the membership, exhorting them to exert their influence in shaping and guiding the trends of the time. He further stated, "The black dentist-citizen-businessman . . . must continue giving of his own time and energies to serve as centers of influence in guiding the destinies of his own community.

"We must not lose our identity or our sense of purpose to serve the public," Dr. Holley concluded, "especially our own generally poor people. Rather, let us help promulgate and administer the laws by which we live."

Chapter IX

The National Dental

Association

Sporadic efforts to organize black dentists took place before the turn of the century, but the dental division of the North State Medical Society of North Carolina (founded in 1887) claims the distinction of being the first such organization.

By 1900 the impact of the X-ray machine (invented in 1895 by Wilhelm Konrad Roentgen) was being felt by both the medical and dental professions. There was great demand for information about this radical aid to diagnosis. Gold, various amalgams, cements, and other filling materials were constantly being improved by manufacturers and members of the profession, and the fusing of porcelain, the casting of gold restorations, and the use of newer local anesthetic agents were also subjects of profound interest. It was critically important to provide this information to all licensed dentists, and the formation of dental societies provided the best method of dissemination.

At this time many dentists were members of established medical societies on an associate basis, or of the dental divisions of such societies. Their specific needs, however, were usually left unfulfilled in medical meetings, where innovations and new discoveries in the field of dentistry were seldom discussed. (This was true despite the fact that in 1867 the Harvard University Medical School recognized the profession by establishing a school of dentistry.) The incorporation of dental divisions into the other nationally prominent medical schools, from 1870 to 1900, has served to rescue a deteriorating profession from public contempt. But acceptance of dentistry as a profession coequal with medicine was withheld — to a great extent by senior physicians' groups.

Because of this negative attitude toward dentists and the exclusion of blacks from the white dental societies, on November 14, 1900, the Washington Society of Colored Dentists was founded, with the hope of eventually establishing a national organization. These efforts were initiated in May of 1901, when D.A. Ferguson of Richmond, Virginia, issued a call for the meeting on July 5, 1901 in Washington, D.C., at the Dental College of Howard University. Dr. Ferguson was elected president of this group and D.W. Onley of Washington was named secretary. Problems of mutual interest and the formation of a national group were discussed. Also, plans were made to catalogue the names of all black dentists in the United States for the permanent archives of the group. In addition, all dentists were informed about the group and the advantages of membership. Committees were organized to effect these, and other plans.

In July, 1902 a second meeting was held in Washington. Papers were presented on prosthesis by several members, and the use of scientific articulators and newer impression techniques were also discussed. The highlight of the session was a paper on orthodontia by Dr. Ferguson. Some dentists rejected the theme of his paper because it offered a plan of treatment black patients were financially unable to afford. (This concern for the low economic status of their clientele produced a certain cohesiveness among the black dentists.) The conditions of black dental colleges were discussed and plans were made to seek financial assistance.

It is noteworthy that problems to which the present NDA addresses itself are essentially the same as those recognized and challenged by these pioneers. The revolutionary steps taken at the 1902 meeting were said by many to have galvanized black dentists into action, an attitude which has persisted throughout the succeeding years of the organization. A determination de-

veloped that neither caste nor any of its frustrating conse-
quences would be allowed to deter black dentists from achieving
professional standing and the same high quality performance
shown by white practitioners.

The third annual meeting was held July 4-6, 1903 in Washington, D.C. The theme was the dissemination of information
revolving around the widespread movement for increased efficiency in the practice. The agenda also included the refinement
of the work of previously appointed committees and new strate-
gies to increase the organization's membership.

The 1905 meeting was the last held by this national society.
However, the Washington Society of Colored Dentists, which
had been associated with the now defunct national organization,
was intensely disappointed by the collapse of the larger movement and more determined than ever to maintain the Washington nucleus of membership. Members of the Society were required to be residents of the District of Columbia. Associate
members, however, lived outside the metropolitan area. All
strove to implement many of the programs of the original national association.

In 1907, the Washington Society of Colored Dentists changed
its name to the Robert Tanner Freeman Dental Society in honor
of a native Washingtonian who, in 1869, became the first black to
receive the D.D.S. degree from Harvard University.

The progress of the Washington Society was observed by
other area dentists. By 1905, the Maryland Dental Society was
founded, and D.A. Ferguson, along with a few other dedicated
colleagues, maintained a strong organization in Virginia.

The twelfth annual banquet of the Washington Society was
held in Baltimore, with dentists from Maryland and Virginia as
guests. The idea of the formation of an organization of black
dentists from the three adjoining localities was the chief topic of
discussion. The motion to organize such a group was passed by
unanimous consent. Designated as committee chairmen to from
the Tri-State Society were Drs. Ferguson and J.M.G. Ramsey.

The notice of the intended meeting for the formation of the
new Society went out in January 1913 to all black dentists in

Maryland, Virginia, and the District of Columbia. The group met at Buckroe Beach, Virginia on July 19, 1913, a date now accepted as the founding date of the National Dental Association (NDA). Among the original members were several pioneer dentists: John E. Washington of Washington, D.C., the first black dentist licensed by the District Board of Dental Examiners in 1905; George H. Butler, first dentist to join the Washington Society of Colored Dentists after its founding in 1903; A.O. Reid and O.D. Jones of Baltimore; and Sumner Wormley, also of Washington.

Essentially, this convention was a social one. However, the purpose of establishing mutual respect and an association of qualified dentists had been accomplished. It should be remembered that this was still a time when large numbers of poorly trained, unscrupulous dentists were commonplace, and the licensing of state dental boards ineffectual. Men who had been in practice prior to the establishment of these boards at the beginning of the century were permitted to continue the practice. The boards, however, controlled the selection and rejection of new dental candidates. Among those already in practice were many who had been trained in the dental school "diploma factories," with little formal education past grammar school. Although some possessed exceptional mechanical ability, others lacked even this basic talent.

During the era of the Tri-State Society's formation, the development of better local anesthetic solutions, the refinement of vaso-constrictors for these solutions, and experimentation with conduction anesthesia were of intense interest to dentists. The demand for the presentation of this new knowledge led to the Society to incorporate scientific sessions into the conventions. Soon, discussions about articulators, anesthesia, general versus local anesthetic agents, and the ethics of professional behavior attracted men from other states to Buckroe Beach. By 1918, just five years after its establishments, Tri-State became the Interstate Dental Association. From 1913 to 1918, the "scientific" sessions were devoted only to the reading and discussion of professional papers, but in 1919, the first clinics were incorporated into the sessions.

Meanwhile, a few dentists of the Interstate Dental Association became affiliated with the dental division of the National Medical Association (NMA). These dentists held their conventions in conjunction with those of physicians and pharmacists throughout the country. Positions of relative importance were held by some dentists within the framework of the NMA. The Association's favorable reputation attracted many dentists, but many physicians and pharmacists as well as dentists were concerned about its limited membership. They felt that unity in numbers was essential to strength.

Generally, the dental division remained a satellite of the NMA, and many dentists resented what they imagined to be a condescending attitude on the part of the physicians. Some dentists felt that their physician confreres fell just short of arrogance. Dissatisfaction with the NMA made membership in the Interstate Dental Association even more appealing. By 1928, fifteen years after the founding of the original Tri-State Society, the roster of its membership was impressive (see Table 4).

In 1930, the Interstate Dental Association met at Buckroe Beach for the last time. The 1931 convention was moved to Howard University by the invitation of Dean Arnold Donawa and the faculty. The intense emphasis upon a scientific program dictated this move to a site where the most satisfactory presentation of live demonstrations was possible. Undoubtedly, the scientific program at Howard and the tone of the convention set a standard of excellence to which the founders of the Association had long aspired. It was decided that rather than return to Buckroe Beach, the next convention would accept the invitation of the Commonwealth Dental Society of New Jersey to meet at Bordertown in 1932. That convention resulted in the establishment of the second national association which, in 1933, adopted a new name: the National Dental Association (NDA). Historically, the American and Southern Dental Associations, founded in 1859 and 1869, respectively, had joined forces in 1897 and assumed the name "National Dental Association," However, in 1922 this joint organization reverted to its original title, the

TABLE 4

INTERSTATE DENTAL ASSOCIATION, 1928

District of Columbia

F. P. Barrier†
J. C. Brazier
Roscoe C. Brown†
George H. Butcher†
Benjamin H. Early
F. D. Edwards
Thomas W. Edwards†
Elias G. Evans
C. C. Fry†
A. E. Gaskins†
Charles S. Godden†
Ernest M. Gould
C. A. Gray†
Vernon S. Green
W. E. Hamilton†
Lee Holton
Q. Bernard King
S. J. Lewis
E. E. T. Mavritte
I. O. Mitchell
Harvey S. Nicholson
A. A. Russell
S. D. Savoy
R. B. Thomas
John A. Turner
R. G. Walker
Adolphus Walton
J. E. Washington†
R. M. West
R. B. M. Wilson†
M. D. Wiseman
C. S. Wormley†

Maryland (1913)*

B. F. Brown, Baltimore
D. C. Brown†, Baltimore
Robert J. Hackett, Baltimore
O. D. Jones†, Baltimore
O. W. McNeil, Annapolis
William B. Mason, Baltimore
A. O. Reid†, Baltimore
Albert A. Smith, Baltimore
Charles E. Watts, Baltimore
Isaac Young, Baltimore

Virginia (1913)*

J.H. Anderson, So. Boston
W. B. Anderson†, Portsmouth
C. R. Ballard, Berkley-Norfolk
L. A. Banks, Newport News
E. E. Bassette, Richmond
R. Beecher, Taylor, Richmond
Richard H. Bland, Suffolk
F. F. Bradley, Berkley-Norfolk
R. J. Brown†, Norfolk
S. D. Calloway, Richmond
James A. Childs, Richmond
John Childs, Staunton
William Coleman, Norfolk
B. A. Coles, Charlottesville
S. F. Coppage, Norfolk
C. S. Cowan, Danville
D. Eugene Dabney, Newport News
E. D. Downing, Roanoke
G. P. Downing, Roanoke
E. R. Dudley, Roanoke
A. F. Evans, Lynchburg
D. A. Ferguson†, Richmond
J. E. Fowlkes, S. Richmond
L. A. Fowlkes, Newport News
J. E. Gary, Danville
W. L. Harris, Fredericksburg
William S. Hart, Hampton
Joshua L. Hartwell, Petersburg
J. A. Jackson, Charlottesville
O. R. Johnson†, Petersburg
W. M. Logan, Petersburg†
W. T. Lovette, Norfolk
J. L. McGriff, Portsmouth
O. W. Marshall, Staunton
Fred Morton, Richmond
W. Pettis, Richmond
E. B. Pressley, Clifton Forge
J. M. G. Ramsey†, Richmond
E. H. L. Ranse†, Suffolk
Edwina M. Reeves, Suffolk
L. A. Reid, Richmond
G. C. Strong†, Norfolk
S. A. Thomas, Newport News
J. M. Tinsley, Richmond
Floyd W. Turner, Portsmouth
M. M. Ward, Newport News
H. P. Weedon, Lynchburg
A. J. Wells, Norfolk
D. B. Williams, Richmond

North Carolina (1915)*

John J. Adams, Fayetteville
J. W. Black, Rocky Mount
F. C. Cook, Elizabeth City
A. L. Cromwell, Winston-Salem
L. Davenport, Henderson
C. A. Dunston, Raleigh
G. G. Evans, Raleigh
W. L. Horne, Weldon
A. S. Hunter, Durham
C. O. Lee, Winston-Salem
W. H. Philips, Wilson
A. W. Rivera, Greensboro
George C. Simkins, Greensboro
E. W. Smith, Winston-Salem

Source: Interstate Dental Association.   *Year of entry   † Deceased

American Dental Association (ADA).

The thirty-third annual convention, the first under the new banner, was hosted by the Odonto-Chirurgical Society of Philadelphia and Sylvester B. Smith, its president. The meeting, which continued from July 10-13, outlined the organizational structure of this new national association and offered surgical clinics.

The 1934 convention, hosted by Meharry Medical College in Nashville, Tennessee, July 9-13, was well attended. Under the direction of President Melancthon D. Wiseman, the scientific content of the program was augmented and the NDA's progress was phenomenal. Yet many members of the dental division of the NMA were not interested in the progress of this substantial, growing association.

During the next two years, despite the previous rift between the two organizations, many physicians of the NMA wished to rejoin forces with the NDA. At the 1936 NDA convention in Louisville, Kentucky, a telegram from the NMA was read which expressed these desires. However, due to the increasing lack of interest within the NMA, the NDA refused to accept the offer. (At this time, NDA membership was approximately 200.)

In 1937, the convention returned to Howard University College of Dentistry in Washington. At that time, Dr. Russell A. Dixon was Dean of the College. Registrations that year totaled 335 as the departure from the NMA dental division increased. With a superb scientific clinic, Jackson L. (Jack) Davis, the president, welcomed visitors with what amounted to a *voup de grace* for the NMA dental division:

> As president, I appeal to the present membership to
> invite all worthy unaffiliated ethical practitioners
> to become members of the association so that the
> benefits accruing from organized dentistry may be shared
> by all. It is my deepest concern that this and each
> succeeding meeting will be a source of educational
> and relaxational benefit to our entire profession.

FIGURE 1

ORGANIZATIONAL STRUCTURE OF THE NATIONAL DENTAL ASSOCIATION, 1968

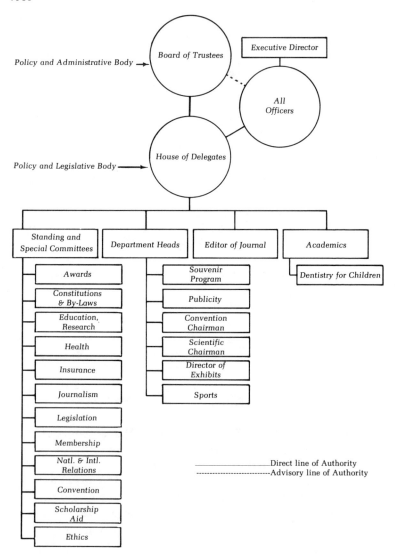

Source: Eddie G. Smith, president, National Dental Association, 1972-73.

The 1939 convention, planned to coincide with the New York World's Fair, met as scheduled in August. Drawing 365 registered dentists, it was marked by excellent scientific sessions, outlined in the souvenir program of some 88 pages which included some of the most interesting tracts and histories yet published in the field. The maturity and stability of the NDA was now assured; black dentists accepted the programming and direction of the organization as professional, discrete, and rewarding. The level of achievement had now been reached that seemed to require only maintenance, hardly renaissance.

The Chicago Convention of 1938, the first of several held in that city, was well attended and well programmed. It was the first NDA convention to be held in the midwest, and strangely enough, marked the initiation of a power struggle within the association which grew to great proportions in ensuing years.

Dentists within the NDA graduated primarily from two colleges, Howard and Meharry. Significant school pride remains with their graduates; some say that the present struggle for political power within the NDA is a direct outgrowth of this very human phenomenon. Traditionally, Meharry graduates tended to practice in the West and South, while Howard graduates were distributed along the Atlantic seaboard. There are notable exceptions, but overall, the same boundaries remain. Attempts by dentists from both groups, principally East vs. South and West, resulted in jockeying for position within the NDA, as it steadily enlarged and became more influential. Dentists within the organization say that the political struggle has had no ill effect upon the success of the NDA, that it functioned as excellently from 1940 to 1963 as it did during the first quarter-century. But others deny this, and state that the association has dragged its feet for some twenty years or more. The 1938 convention marked the turning point toward a more peaceful coexistence of the contending groups, and the NDA since then has selected its executives strictly on merit rather than because of personal popularity.

Since its inception, the NDA performed commendably as an instrument of black dentistry in the field of civil rights. In 1937, for example, the Association pressed for enactment of a bill for the District of Columbia (as hundreds of dentists encountered prejudice in the capital during the NDA convention). Also in that same year, the NDA supported a bill to increase the number of dentists in the Army and Navy. During the 1930s, the NDA also supported a bill to provide financial assistance to families unable to afford the rising costs of medical treatment.

The first year of the second half-century of the NDA — 1964 — was marked with increased legal activity in the area of civil rights. An all-out assault was waged on racial segregation and discrimination to insure the right of every qualified black dentist to become a member of the ADA and all of its component societies. In 1964 and the following years, black dentists became members of state dental associations in Texas, Georgia, North

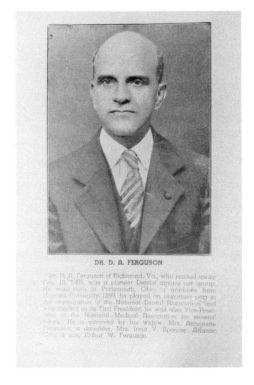

DR. D. A. FERGUSON

Dr. D. A. Ferguson of Richmond, Va., who passed away Feb. 10, 1935, was a pioneer Dentist among our group. He was born in Portsmouth, Ohio, a graduate from Howard University 1899, he played an important part in the organization of the National Dental Association and was elected as its First President, he was also Vice-President of the National Medical Association for several years. He is survived by his widow, Mrs. Antoinette Ferguson, a daughter, Mrs. Irma V. Spencer, Atlantic City, a son, Arthur W. Ferguson.

Dr. D.A. Ferguson, a pioneering member of the National Dental Association, was the organization's first president.

Carolina, Virginia, Louisiana, and Tennessee. (In 1964, the NDA also produced its first film on preventive dentistry, "Happy Teeth — Happy Smile." The second film, "Teeth Are for Life," was produced in 1967.)

The Ladies Auxiliary of the NDA was organized August 6, 1936, in Cincinnati, Ohio, for the purpose of creating interest in and stimulating attendance at the annual meetings. The activities were predominantly social at first, but have expanded to include programs and projects more germane to the profession.

Across the nation, auxiliaries have undertaken the task of forming dental career clubs in high schools and some colleges based on the theme "Mobilizing Youth for Dental Careers." The focus is on tenth, eleventh, and twelfth grade students and college freshmen. The clubs use films, field trips to dental facilities, lectures and forums to disseminate information to young people on the vast areas and resources available to them in the field. Scholarships and other awards are an important part of the program.

The auxiliary contributed funds to the National Council of Negro Women toward the establishment of a Memorial Park in Washington, D.C., honoring Mary McLeod Bethune, founder of Bethune-Cookman College, Daytona Beach, Florida (1904), and director of the Negro Affairs Division of the National Youth Administration under President Franklin D. Roosevelt.

The Auxiliary's publication, The Standard, is published annually. (The present editor is Amanda Ruth Smith of Dallas, Texas.)

Table 5
NATIONAL DENTAL ASSOCIATION PRESIDENTS

President	Year	Location
D. A. Ferguson	1913-18	Richmond, Virginia
C. A. Dunston	1918-20	Raleigh, North Carolina
S. J. Lewis	1920-22	Manassas, Virginia
J. M. G. Ramsey	1922-23	Richmond, Virginia
I. M. Lawrence	1923-24	Philadelphia, Pennsylvania

NATIONAL DENTAL ASSOCIATION PRESIDENTS (continued)

President	Year	Location
W. B. Reed	1924-26	Nashville, Tennessee
G. H. Butcher	1926-28	Washington, D.C.
A. O. Reid	1928-29	Baltimore, Maryland
H. A. McAllister	1929-30	Hampton, Virginia
E. D. Downing	1930-32	Roanoke, Virginia
D. A. Ferguson	1932-33	Richmond, Virginia
M. D. Wiseman	1933-34	Washington, D.C.
C. W. Dorsey	1934-35	Philadelphia, Pennsylvania
W. B. Reed	1935-36	Nashville, Tennessee
J. L. Davis	1936-37	Washington, D.C.
R. E. Beaman	1937-38	Cincinnati, Ohio
S. C. Hamilton	1938-39	Chicago, Illinois
W. J. Howard	1939-40	Houston, Texas
J. L. Baxter	1940-41	Orange, New Jersey
L. A. Reid	1941-42	Richmond, Virginia
W. O. Claytor	1942-44	Washington, D.C.
D. H. Turpin	1944-46	Nashville, Tennessee
R. H. Thompson	1946-47	Westfield, New Jersey
E. W. Taggert	1947-48	Birmingham, Alabama
R. A. Dixon	1948-49	Washington, D.D.
W. D. Giles	1949-50	Chicago, Illinois
M. L. Walton	1950-51	Thomasville, Georgia
W. M. Springer	1951-52	Cincinnati, Ohio
A. M. Mackel	1952-53	Natchez, Mississippi
C. L. Thomas	1953-54	Louisville, Kentucky
J. E. Carter, Jr.	1954-55	Augusta, Georgia
J. E. Bowman	1955-56	Washington, D.C.
L. W. R. Gates	1956-57	Darby, Pennsylvania
H. T. Penn	1957-58	Roanoke, Virginia
C. E. Williams	1958-59	Chicago, Illinois
H. M. Proffitt	1959-60	Helena, Arkansas
W. H. A. Elliott	1960-61	Huntington, West Virginia
J. B. Singleton	1961-62	Nashville, Tennessee
R. Layne	1962-63	St. Louis, Missouri
M. Mitchell	1964-65	Washington, D.C.
W. J. Walker	1965-66	Chicago, Illinois
H. R. Primas, Jr.	1966-67	Pittsburgh, Pennsylvania
J. A. A. Catchings	1967-68	Detroit, Michigan
F. Chowning	1968-69	Indianapolis, Indiana
J. W. Holly	1969-70	Portsmouth, Virginia

NATIONAL DENTAL ASSOCIATION PRESIDENTS (continued)

President	Year	Location
C. Broadus	1970-71	Fort Worth, Texas
R. Smith	1971-72	Daytona Beach, Florida
E. G. Smith	1972-73	Washington, D.C.
M. W. Roseman	1973-74	Cleveland, Ohio
Frank Shuford	1974-75	Washington, D.C.
Charles Williams	1975-76	Chicago, Illinois
Harvey Webb, Jr.	1976-77	Baltimore, Maryland

Source: National Dental Association.

Chapter X

Black Membership in the

American Dental

Association

The color line in American dentistry has faded officially into oblivion and has been relegated at last to its place in history. The question of race no longer appears on application blanks of component and constituent societies of the ADA, rosters of state boards, dental schools, and dental organizations. By-laws have been changed to delete all references to race, creed, and color, and black dentists hold offices, chair committees, and enjoy complete membership privileges in all dental associations. As a direct result of the eradication of these membership restrictions, black dentists now serve on state boards of dental examiners, dental school faculties, hospital staffs, attend seminars and conventions, and enjoy the fraternization that ensues from these relationships. Furthermore, mutual instruction, protection, support, and encouragement are engendered by these associations.

To become a member of the ADA, a dentist must first be accepted as a member of a component local society, unless he or she is a member of one of the federal dental services. To become a member of a component society, the dentist must meet the following qualifications:

1. be a graduate of an accredited school or college of dentistry;

2. be licensed to practice;
3. have completed the membership application form;
4. agree to adhere to a code of dental ethics.

Some societies request sponsorship by one or two members, but this is a routine consideration and not a binding condition.

Membership in the ADA has not always been simple or routine for black dentists in several of the Southern states—a fact well known but for long ignored by those holding official positions in dentistry. To become a member of an official dental organization, a private practitioner must hold membership at each of the society's three levels: local, state, and national. Black dentists have been refused membership at the local level in the South, thereby aborting all chances of enjoying the benefits of the national organization.

It was not until the 103rd annual convention of the ADA that the question of black membership received serious attention by that body. An editorial in the *Journal* stated, "At the 1962 annual session held in Miami Beach, the House of Delegates, by a near unanimous vote, adopted a resolution which will ease the way for all qualified Negro dentists to become members of the American Dental Association and all of its component and constituent societies." This action was a result of a 1958 resolution of the National Dental Association requesting the ADA "to consider the sponsorship of resolutions urging constituent, component and state societies having racially restrictive membership provisions to restudy these with a view towards eliminating them."

Prior to 1958 black dentists in Washington, D.C., the Nation's Capital, could not join the ADA. Even the dean of the Meharry School of Dentistry was not eligible for membership because of the racially restrictive clauses in the Tennessee society's by-laws.

At the 1960 session, the Board of Trustees stated that "the ADA and its constituent and component societies are established to make the benefits of professional organizations available to members of the profession. The Board of Trustees, therefore, requests that the constituent and component societies study their by-laws with a view to insuring that there are no provisions which restrict membership on the basis of race, creed, or color."

Hence, in 1962 the following Resolution was adopted by a nearly unanimous vote:

> 71-1962-B. Resolved, that the By-laws, Chapter V, House of Delegates, Section 30F—Powers, be amended by the addition of the following sentence: "It shall also have the power to suspend the representation for a constituent society in the House of Delegates upon a determination by the House that the By-laws of the constituent society violate the Constitution of By-laws of this Association."

Prior to this action, the only course the ADA had to follow, in areas where constituent by-laws were in conflict with the by-laws of the national association, was the suspension or revocation of a charter. The ADA preferred not to take this course of action and sought other means to impose sanctions on those societies in violation. Thus, on November 1, 1962 the House of Delegates passed the now historic resolution amending its own by-laws with the stipulation "that a vote refusing to seat a delegation must pass by a two-thirds majority and the society must be given a year's warning time."

This action was followed by a timely editorial in the December 1962 issue of the *Journal,* "Membership of Negroes in the American Dental Association," which stated in part:

> This commendable action [the resolution] is in keeping with the wording and the intent of Article Two of the Association's Constitution. The object of the Association shall be to encourage the improvement of the health of the public and to promote the art and science of dentistry . . . The denial of membership in the association to qualified dentists on the basis of race, creed, or color, aborts the object of the association, because such discriminatory policies impede the professional growth of all dentists and, therefore work to the detriment of the public welfare.

Many white dentists and organizations were then free to act on behalf of their fellow dentists denied these basic rights. Jay Wolff of Oxon Hill, Maryland, wrote the editor of the *Journal* (in June 1963) to complain that "a lamentable condition was allowed to exist by the ADA by either ignoring it completely or treating it with smug self-interest and hypocrisy." Speaking of the discrimination within its ranks, he continued: "This is a moral and professional disgrace to ourselves and our organization. The American Dental Association should be for all American dentists, and the time is long past due for us to make it so."

The February 6, 1964 edition of the Atlanta *Constitution* printed the following statement: "The Georgia Dental Association's statutory right to nominate members of certain state boards make it unconstitutional for it to exclude Negroes from its membership, according to a federal court ruling."

U.S. District Court Judge Frank A. Hooper did not order the Association to do anything but to obey these stated objectives when he denied the Association's motion to dismiss a suit by black dentist R. C. Bell of Atlanta, which stated that excluding blacks "seems to be a clear violation of the equal protection clause" of the Constitution.[1]

Except for the acts of the Georgia legislature which require appointments to the State Board of Health, the Board of Dental Examiners, and the Hospital Advisory Council to be made from nominees submitted by the national association, the Georgia Dental Association and the Northern District Dental Society would have the unquestioned right to admit only such persons as they desired and, without violating any law, could exclude blacks from membership.

The Georgia legislature, however, by giving the state dental association the right to nominate members to the three state agencies referred to in this action, made it an agency of the State of Georgia, Hooper declared.

This case denied black dentists equal protection of the Constitutional laws because they were thereby deprived of the right to vote on the members of the association who, as board members, enacted the rules under which they practiced and licensed dentists.

Judge Hooper originally signed an order on January 21 deny-
ing the state dental association's motion to dismiss the suit. At
the request of the association, and with the concurrence of the
plaintiffs, he later voided that order and issued another with the
same conclusions, specifying that it could be appealed to the
Fifth Circuit Court on interlocutory appeal.

On June 19, 1964, U.S. District Judge Wilson Warlick dis-
missed a suit brought by Reginald A. Hawkins of Charlotte, who
sought to enjoin the North Carolina Dental Society and the
Second District Dental Society from barring him from membership on alleged racial grounds. Judge Warlick ruled that the two
societies had not violated Hawkins's constitutional rights.

Hawkins immediately took the case to the U.S. Court of
Appeals in Richmond, Virginia, to strike down discriminatory
policies of the North Carolina Dental Society. NAACP Legal
Defense Fund Attorneys, acting on Dr. Hawkins's, behalf, told
the Appeals Court that the "numerous activities of the North
Carolina Dental Society made it a dominant force in regulating
dentistry" in the state.

The *Journal* of the California Dental Association noted the
verdict against Hawkins in an editorial in October 1964:

> This Judge has used our most sacred document of justice
> the Constitution of the United States, to skirt justice and
> to find a refuge for injustice. May the Supreme Court of
> the United States reverse his decision unanimously. Only
> this will restore my faith in American justice.

On February 16, 1965, the Board of Trustees of the Eleventh
District Dental Society of New York unanimously approved the
following resolution:

> *Whereas:* The background statement presented clearly
> denotes exclusions from membership in the American
> Dental Association, constituent and component societies
> of North Carolina, of Negro dentists eminently qualified
> by reason of licensure, practice, citizenship, and

character, and whereas: Membership in the American Dental Association (predicated upon prior membership in constituent dental societies) is, in North Carolina, in fact denied all qualified Negro applicants solely on the basis of color, and

Whereas: In 1961, the American Dental Association directed all constituent and component societies to insure that their by-laws contained no provision which discriminated against candidates for membership on the basis of race, creed or color (ADA Transactions, 1961), pp. , and whereas: The actions related to Dr. Hawkins and others who have applied for membership and have been arbitrarily denied solely because they are Negro completely negate the intent and purpose of the resolution and directive of the American Dental Association, and

Whereas: The Board of Trustees of the American Dental Association *(ADA Transactions 1962,* pgs. 343-344) has approved its committee's report that, "it is obvious that provisions not expressed in constituent or component society bylaws are being enforced to compel discrimination on the basis of race, creed or color" and "that these unconstitutional procedures of constituent and component societies not sanctioned by their by-laws have not yet been challenged". . . . and

Whereas: The Civil action of Dr. Hawkins versus the North Carolina Dental Society *et al,* now constitutes a challenge to the abuses evident in the unconstitutional exclusion of Negro dentists from membership,

Therefore: The Eleventh District Dental Society hereby resolves and respectfully petitions the Dental Society of the State of New York to submit to the 1965 annual meeting of the American Dental Association the following resolution:

Resolved: That the Dental Society of the State of New York, in agreement with the American Dental Association Board of Trustees, deems it essential "to eliminate the allegation that it is tacitly cooperating with restrictive practices by constituent and component societies, which, in reality, do discriminate in membership entrance on the basis of race, creed or color" and petitions the American Dental Association to take resolute action to enforce the actual intent of its 1961 resolution to prevent discrimination in membership entrance on the basis of race, creed or color, and:

1. to advise all constituent and component societies that nonconformance with the spirit and the intent as well as the letter of the ADA by-laws may lead to sanctions provided, including revocation of charter;
2. to encourage all members of the National Dental Association not enrolled in the American Dental Association to submit applications for membership;
3. seeing to it that the 1961 statement of the American Dental Association with regard to discrimination in constituent and component society by-laws is intended to insure that no local subterfuge (such as inability to obtain sponsoring signatures) will allow such discrimination.

The Bulletin of the Eleventh District Dental Society of New York State (March-April 1965, Vol. 3, No. 3) discussed the Hawkins case and concluded the following:

1. Dr. Hawkins deserves personal praise and support for courage.
2. The Hawkins case deserves support organizationally. The ADA should be requested, through the usual channels of organization, to enforce the letter and spirit of the 1961 resolution. All qualified dentists must have the right to belong.
3. The ADA through its leadership and Journal should educate its members as to the fundamental social

issues involved and exercise a moral force in a
forthright manner.

4. Our members should express their views by means
of a letter-to-the-editor of ADA, and to our delegates to
the ADA.

5. Those members who have professional friends in
the South—white dentists—should communicate with
them and encourage them to support the Negro
dentists who will be coming forward more and more to
obtain membership.

The April 1965 issue of the ADA *Journal* reported that Fred-
erick Kraus, a white professor of dentistry at the University of
Alabama and former chief of dental service at the VA Hospital in
Birmingham, said that after twelve years of silence on the civil
rights issue, his conscience had forced him to take a public
stand. He joined a new group known as Concerned White Citizens of Alabama, which staged its first demonstration during the
Selma crisis: "We have remained silent for a long time trying to
give moral support to the Negroes; we have waited for changes
and improvements but nothing changes and nothing improves. I
personally felt it was time to show that a group of demonstrators
can have a face other than that of a Negro. I feel what we did will
give more white citizens the courage to stand up for equality for
both Negroes and whites." Kraus added that he had no fear of
losing his job.

Finally, at the May 15, 1965 meeting of the North Carolina
Dental Society, the House of Delegates voted to repeal the provisions of the by-laws which prevented black dentists from membership and to which the ADA's Board of Trustees had strongly
objected.

In 1966, the U.S. Court of Appeals for the Fourth Circuit
reversed a federal district court decision and ordered that court
to hold further proceedings in the Hawkins case. In reversing the
decision, the appeals court noted that only as a member of the
ADA could a professionally qualified, licensed dentist have a
voice in elections and appointments to staff offices filled by

dentists.

Reginald A. Hawkins finally was accepted as a member of the Second District Dental Society, the North Carolina Dental Society, and the American Dental Association in 1966, after his case had cost the NAACP Legal Defense Fund over $24,000 and four years of litigation.

This was, undoubtedly, the most expensive membership fee ever "assessed." But the cost, in terms of dollars-and-cents, was not the only consideration. A myriad of delaying tactics, subterfuges and outright rejections without cause or explanation previously had blocked the paths of many black dentists trying to gain admittance to the ADA.

The September 20, 1965 Greensboro *Record* carried the following story:

> Three Negro dentists here were notified by the Third District Dental Society that their application for membership had been denied. The dentists are W. L. T. Miller, B. W. Barnes, and George C. Simkins, Jr. All three dentists have practiced here a number of years, Dr. Barnes over 40 years. Dr. Miller and Dr. Barnes were denied on second application, having been turned down for membership a year ago. Dr. Simkins was making his first application for membership.
>
> Dr. Simkins said that no reason was given for the rejections, which came by telegram.

Some border states did not wait for definitive directives from the ADA and accepted blacks for membership as early as 1956 (Oklahoma) and 1958 (Washington D.C., and Kansas City, Missouri). Kentucky accepted blacks for the first time in 1959. Societies in the deep South, however, did not capitulate until the early 1960s, and only then after much prodding by the parent organization.

In April 1961, black dentists in New Orleans, Memphis, Dallas, Atlanta, Houston, and Miami attended scientific sessions with white dentists for the first time at a closed circuit television clinic sponsored by the Proctor and Gamble Company, and then only because the ADA insisted that black dentists be invited to the showings.

In the meantime, the NDA was pursuing with great vigor its "Operation: Membership" program, initiated a few years earlier. C. O. Simpkins, ardent chairman of the Civil Rights Committee for the NDA, urged all black dentists to apply for membership in the ADA through their local and state societies and recommended that the NDA send an open letter to the ADA "requiring a speed-up of remunerative action and discontinuance of all subterfuge." He further stated that the ADA had informed this (Civil Rights) committee that questionnaires had been sent to all societies in order to determine what action they had taken to comply with the decisions of the Board of Trustees to eliminate discrimination against Negro dentists applying for membership in constituent and component societies.

The Comittee was further informed that the results had not been tabulated and a report on the questionnaires would be presented to the Board of Trustees which met August 24-27, 1966. "In our inquiry as to the action taken on the affidavits stating the denial of Negro dentists as members, we were informed that they imagine the affidavits will be considered by the Board (ADA) at that time," Dr. Simpkins stated.

"Affidavits," Dr. Simpkins continued," are still being received from our colleagues who are blatantly refused membership in their societies. Progress is slow and sometimes not at all. With dentistry reaching new horizons and the advent of Medicare programs, this negative progress is strangulation and stagnation."

Emil W. Lentchner, a member of the state Board of Governors of the New York Dental Society and delegate of the ADA, addressed the NDA at its fifty-third annual convention in August 1966 on this subject and seriously questioned the statistics culled from questionnaires. "After all," he stated, "a 100 percent increase in membership of Negro dentists in some Southern states is an increase from one-to-two. And the fact that all states except Missouri now have at least one Negro member does not indicate any but token compliance." Dr. Lentchner made the following suggestions for immediate action by the NDA:

1. That letters be written to Drs. Gardner and Quigley of HEW, reminding them of the fine observations and sincere concerns they expressed, and reporting that nine months after the resolutions, there had been nothing to denote any positive progress to end discriminatory practices. A request for a conference with HEW was indicated.

2. The NDA should request a hearing before the Board of Trustees meeting in August, to express its concerns that the 1965 resolutions were not being swiftly and firmly implemented.

3. The following open letter to the Board of Trustees of the ADA should be published:

To the Board of Trustees–American Dental Association

We agree that discrimination in membership practices must be eliminated. We declare our unqualified support for the resolutions passed by the House of Delegates of the American Dental Association in Las Vegas in November 1965.

Especially do we applaud the proposed mechanism in Report No. 7 of the Board of Trustees designed to implement declared policy of the American Dental Association to end discrimination within its ranks. We agree that the words are heartening.

Our concerns are highlighted by events since November which include the dastardly bombing of the home of Dr. Hawkins and the continuing resistance of some segments to expressions for integration.

Our concerns are accented by the silence of the Board of Trustees since the commendable policy statements in Report No. 7.

Documented complaints of discrimination in membership policies have been filed.

We ask you to demonstrate without equivocation—that the ADA means what it says.

We ask you to implement the fine declarations of November with equally fine action—NOW!

We ask you to insure that equality in membership becomes a reality, not merely a theory.

It is some nine months since the Las Vegas resolutions. Discrimination in membership practices flagrantly continues as if those declarations had never been made.

At the March 1966 meeting of the Executive Board, the Committee on Civil Rights requested that the following copy of a blank affidavit be published in the *Quarterly* of the NDA with a request to apply immediately for membership in the local, state, and national dental associations. The affidavits and other related information were to be mailed to Dr. Cuthbert Simpkins, chairman, Civil Rights Committee, NDA

AFFIDAVIT

STATE OF _____
COUNTY OF _____
NAME _____ being first duly sworn, according to law, deposes and says:

1. I am a citizen of the United States and the State of _____ residing in _____ County or Parish. My present address is _____ State.
2. I have resided at the above address since _____ .
3. I meet the qualifications established by the Constitution and By-Laws of the American Dental Association for membership in its State and Local Dental Societies.
4. I believe that I have been denied the right to membership by the _____ which is a (component or constituent) of the American Dental Association, solely because I am a Negro.
5. On _____ , 19_____ , I applied for admission to the Dental Society of _____ . I was refused membership and the circumstances involving my application and refusal are these:

Signed: _____

Sworn to and subscribed before me this _____ day of _____ , 19____ .

_____
Notary Public

During the next two years—1967 and 1968—the leadership of the NDA continued its unrelenting vigilance on "Operation: Membership." Top-level conferences were held at every opportunity and the subject of ADA membership was given agenda priority at every NDA-ADA Liaison Committee meeting.

With the admission of E. J. Stringer of Columbus, Mississippi (Appendix J) to the ADA, blacks in every state in the Union could now enter the mainstream of American dentistry. Officially, the doors were opened, but James W. Holley, III, who succeeded James Wallace as president of the NDA, felt it necessary to continue to support and expand the activities of the "Committee to End Discrimination in the Dental Profession." "This Committee," Dr. Holley stated, "has provided a central agency whereby moral persuasion and personal commitment of members of organized dentistry have been heard and directed toward the eradication of discrimination in our profession."

Clyde R. Broadus, who succeded Holley, told the Board of Trustees:

> . . . discrimination still exists within the American Dental Association. After five years of struggle, civil rights legislation and all the efforts of numerous well-meaning and conscientious members of the American Dental Association, after the extensive research and presentation by National Dental Association officials, and members of the Committee, to end discrimination, the basic premises as related in 1965 are still being violated by the constituent societies of the American Dental Association and are ample reason for the continued existence and growth of the National Dental Association, if for no other reason than that of guardian of Human Rights.
>
> No American dentist worth his salt can be proud of the progress that this Liaison Comittee is making in correcting the past. In this regard, I feel a high degree of urgency that we continue to take the initiative and bring an end to the racial discrepancies in organized dentistry in the 1970s.

With the problems of black membership in the ADA behind it, or at least in proper perspective, the National Dental Association turned its attention to problems of broader scope of national interest, i.e. health care for the poor.

In another open letter to the membership, Holley stated the following:

> As we enter into the decade of the seventies many of the dental problems which have plagued mankind since time immemorial are still with us. I might note that dental problems are directly linked with a host of serious health, social, psychological, and nutrition problems and the old priorities in dental health must be reordered. The dental problems we face today require a more efficient use of limited resources and a renewed commitment to reach higher national levels of dental health.
>
> Existing poverty among black people intensifies neglect, with dental diseases most prevalent. Compared to the average child, children from low-income families have five times the number of untreated decayed teeth. Many of these poor children are not even examined—much less treated—by a dentist.
>
> These facts prevail despite America's envied world leadership in dental competence. The gap between promise and performance exists not only because we lack professional knowledge or ability. The gap exists largely because we have failed to apply fully the scientific prevention and treatment knowledge we have, because we have failed to develop adequate distribution and financial systems to overcome delivery problems, and because we have not produced a sufficient supply of dental manpower.
>
> All of these problems must be better managed if we as providers are willing to meet the challenges that confront the profession. It is certain that black dentists will continue their active role in meeting this challenge. It's a new year, a new decade, only thirty years shy of a millennium—a good time to start crossing boundaries. A good time to take a chance.

Chapter XI

Selection and Appointment of Black Dentists

to State Boards

of Dental Examiners

Historical Sketch

The statutory law which regulates the dentist's relationship with his state is known as the Dental Practice Act. The Dental Practice Act provides for the creation of a State Board of Dental Examiners, an administrative agency empowered to regulate the practice of dentistry. This accomplished primarily by:

1. setting standards for minimum competence to practice;
2. cooperating in the development of educational programs;
3. developing standards and systems for licensing;
4. administering disciplinary proceedings against violators of statutory rules.

The duties and powers of state dental boards are essentially the same in most jurisdictions, but an examination of each state's Dental Practice Act reveals differences in degrees of power vested in the boards. Notwithstanding these differences, all boards are concerned with the protection of the public from incompetent or unethical practitioners. Protection of the public has been their first priority since Alabama, the first state to enact legislation regulating the practice of dentistry, created a state board in 1841. In 1868 Kentucky passed its law regulating dental practice and, between 1868 and 1876, New York, Ohio, Georgia, New

Table 6

METHODS OF SELECTION AND APPOINTMENT OF MEMBERS OF BOARDS OF DENTISTRY

How Appointed	Number of States
Appointed by governor	8
Appointed by governor from list recommended by state dental society or association	11
Appointed by governor; may be selected from list recommended by state dental society or association	8
Appointed by governor with advice and consent of state senate; may be recommended by state dental society or association	4
Appointed by governor with advice and consent of state senate; may be selected from names recommended by state dental society or association	2
Appointed by governor; state dental society or association may submit recommendations; if so, governor must appoint from society recommendation	2
Appointed by governor; confirmation by state legislature	1
Elected by state dentists	2
Elected by dentists in local district with board vacancy	1
Appointed by governor from nominees selected by dentists in congressional district with board vacancy	1
Appointed by governor from nominees selected by dentists in local district with board vacancy	2
Appointed by governor with advice and consent of council	1
Appointed by governor with advice and consent of the council from recommendations by state dental society	1
Appointed by governor; nominees elected by dentists in congressional district and recommended by board to governor	1
Appointed by governor; state dental association recommends three names to director of department of registration, who selects one and submits nominee's name to governor	1
Appointed by board of commissioners from list recommended by state dental society	1
Appointed by governor with advice from secretary of health and mental hygiene, from state dental association list	1
Appointed by board of regents from commissioner's list	1

Source: B. J. Crawford, secretary/treasurer, American Association of Dental Examiners, Chicago, Illinois, 1976.

Jersey, and Pennsylvania followed.

Selection and Appointment

The number of persons selected to serve on state boards and the manner of selection and appointment vary from state to state. (see Table 6.) Also the term of board appointments varies from three to six years. Some states have nondentists or public members on their boards. California has had public members on the board for many years. Bills were introduced in the Oregon legislature in the mid-1970s to provide for public members. Maryland appointed a dental hygienist to the board in 1975. New Jersey also has two public members. By adding non-practicing members, public participation is assured and criticism of the boards as being too professionally oriented is avoided. In recent years, the ethnic makeup of boards has been further broadened by the appointment of black members.

Black Examiners

Black dentists have been members of state dental boards since 1956 when Walter B. Garvin was appointed to serve in the District of Columbia, thus marking a new era of black participation in the mainstream of American dentistry.

In January 1976, Dr. Foster Kidd queried all fifty-two dental boards about their inclusion of black dentists. One of the questions the survey asked was: Have you ever had a black dentist on your Board of Examiners, and if so, what was the date of first appointment?

The results are shown in Table 7. Twenty-eight jurisdictions responded with fifteen states replying in the affirmative. Washington, D.C. is the only jurisdiction having more than one black serving at the same time. The boards that did not respond to the questionnaire were presumed to have no blacks at the time of the survey. Also, it was noted that some states that responded negatively did not have any black practitioners. Washington, D.C. led in tenure in 1976. Clarence O. Lewis, Jr., had served sixteen

Table 7
BLACK APPOINTEES TO STATE BOARDS OF DENTISTRY IN THE UNITED STATES AND ITS TERRITORIES
THROUGH 1976

State	Appointee	Date of Appointment	Office	Comments
Alabama	None			No response
Alaska	Joshua J. Wright	1965-70	Chairman of dental examiners board, 1967-68	
Arizona	None			No response
Arkansas	None			No response
California	Jack L. Kimbrough Henry Lucas, Jr.	1965-69	President, 1976	
Colorado	None			
Connecticut	None			
Delaware	None			No black dentists registered with board
District of Columbia	Walter B. Garvin	July 1956-Jan. 57		First black dentist appointed to a state board of dentistry
	Clarence O. Lewis, Jr.	Mar. 57-June 73	Secy.-D.C. Board, 1968	Longest tenure of any black board member
	William K. Collins Arnett A. Anderson	June 67-present Oct. 69-present	Secy., 1973-1974	
Florida	Edgar Cosby	1973-present	Secy.-treasurer 1975-1976	

BLACK APPOINTEES TO STATE BOARDS OF DENTISTRY (continued)

State	Appointee	Date of Appointment	Office	Comments
Georgia	Robert Jordan	1973-present		
Hawaii	None			No response
Idaho	None			No black dentist has ever applied or taken Idaho board examination
Illinois	Silas P. Jones	1974-present		
Indiana	Paul A. Stevens	1975-present		
Iowa	None			No response
Kansas	None			
Kentucky	None			
Louisiana	None			
Maine	None			
Michigan	Joe A. Rhinehart	1970-71 (partial term) 1971-present		Reappointed in 1971 for term expiring 1977
Maryland	Sidney O. Burnett	1970-present	President, 1972-73	
Massachusetts	None			No response
Minnesota	None			No response
Mississippi	None			No response
Missouri	None			No response

State	Name	Years	Notes
Montana	None		No response
Nebraska	None		No response
Nevada	James McMillan	1971-present	
New Hampshire	None		
New Jersey	Walter L. Alexander	1972-75	
	Kenneth Butler	1975-present	
New Mexico	None		no response
North Carolina	None		No response
North Dakota	None		No response
Ohio	Robert B. Ford	1974-present	
New York	None		No response
Oklahoma	None		No black dentist has sought office of board member
Oregon	None		No response
Pennsylvania	Edmund B. Priesley	1970-74	Resigned due to ill health in 1974
	Sidney Bridges	1975	
Rhode Island	None		No response
South Carolina	None		No response
South Dakota	None		No response
Tennessee	Eugene S. Kilgore	1976	Tennessee Dental Association nominated black dentist in 1976

BLACK APPOINTEES TO STATE BOARDS OF DENTISTRY (continued)

State	Appointee	Date of Appointment	Office Held	Comments
Texas	Foster Kidd	1973	2nd Vice Pres., 1975 1st Vice Pres., 1976 Pres.-elect, 1977 Pres., 1978	
Utah	None			
Vermont	None			
Virginia	Walter S. Claytor	1970-75	Secy.-Treasurer-1974	No black dentist appointed after Claytor
Washington	None			No response
West Virginia	None			No response
Wisconsin	None			No response
Wyoming	None			No response
Puerto Rico	None			No response

Source: Dr. Foster Kidd, *Quarterly of the National Dental Association,* vol. 35, no. 1, October, 1976.

years. Dr. William K. Collins and Dr. Arnett A. Anderson have served nine and seven years, respectively. These terms of service all indicated reappointments—the rewards of a job well done. Another black to be reappointed was Joe A. Rhinehart of Detroit, Michigan. Dr. Rhinehart was appointed to the Michigan Board in 1970 to complete the unexpired term of a white dentist. In 1971, he was reappointed to serve a full term.

The decade of the seventies witnessed the greatest upsurge in black appointments, an indication that more will probably follow. Although most state governors appoint from a list of nominees supplied by the state dental association, still dominated by whites, the 1976 list of nominees submitted by the Tennessee State Dental Association to the governor included the name of one black dentist.

Black board members have earned the respect of their white counterparts, as evidenced by their election to state board offices. Blacks are serving or have served in every capacity of elected office, from secretary to president of the board. This feeling of mutual understanding, respect, and cordiality also exists at the national level.

William F. Collins of Washington, D.C., was elected president of the American Association of Dental Examiners (AADE) in October 1975, the first black president in its ninety-four year history. This organization, composed of the fifty-two state dental boards, was formed in 1882, when six states banded together to discuss methods of solving their mutual problems. The purpose of the AADE is to assist dental boards in administering to the needs of the dental profession in its various jurisdictions, by exchanging information and engaging in programs and joint activities that deal with the education of professionals, including monitoring the accreditation of schools, colleges, and continuing education programs, and improving the reciprocal relations between jurisdictions. Furthermore, the AADE provides interprofessional communications and engages in activities the jurisdictions determine to be necessary to improve the dental services for the welfare and protection of the general public.

In 1966, there were only three black dental examiners in the

United States. Today, there are approximately fifteen blacks, an increase of almost 500 percent (see Table 8). The total number of black examiners is likely to grow at an even faster rate in the future, as black dentists are now actively seeking nomination to examining boards.

Table 8
BLACK DENTAL EXAMINERS, 1976

State	Name
Alaska	Joshua J. Wright* 1033 W. Fireweed Lane Anchorage 99503
California	Jack J. Kimbrough* 245 25th Street San Diego 92102
	Henry Lucas, Pres. 45 Castro Street, Suite 202 San Francisco 94114
District of Columbia	Clarence O. Lewis* 717 Forida Avenue, N.W. Washington 20001
	William K. Collins 4645 Deane Avenue, N.E. Washington 20019
	Arnette A. Anderson 635 G Street, S.W. Washington 20024
Florida	Edgar Cosby, Secy.,-Treas. 635 N.W. 6th Street Gainesville 32601
Georgia	Robert Jordan 970 Hunter Street, Suite 301 Atlanta 30314
Illinois	Silas P. Jones 4700 Martin Luther King Drive Chicago 60615
Indiana	Paul A. Stevens 2200 Grant Street Gary 46404
Michigan	Joe A. Rhinehart 9141 Dexter Boulevard Detroit 48201

BLACK DENTAL EXAMINERS, 1976 (continued)

State	Name
Maryland	Sidney O. Burnett 1318 N. Caroline Street Baltimore 21213
Nevada	James McMillan 2300 Rancho Drive Las Vegas 89102
New Jersey	Walter L. Alexander* 555 Center Street South Orange 07079
	Kenneth Butler 2357 Union Avenue Pennsauken
Ohio	Robert B. Ford 3807 West Third Dayton 54517
Pennsylvania	Edward B. Priestley* 1512 Overington Street Philadelphia 19124
	Sidney Bridges 945 W. 40th Street Philadelphia 19104
Tennessee	Eugene S. Kilgore 802 Buffalo Street Johnson City 37601
Texas	Foster Kidd, Pres.-elect 1420 Forest Avenue Dallas 75215
Virginia	Walter S. Claytor 413 Gainsboro Road, N.W. Roanoke 24016

Source: American Association of Dental Examiners.

*Past Board Member

Several important questions had to be answered before proposing black nominees. The first related to membership in the state dental associations, which traditionally had not been open to blacks and efforts to join had previously been unsuccessful. Yet, as shown in Chapter X, state membership in these associations is a must for all who aspire to the AADE. Secondly, the politics associated with appointments to state agencies is a factor, since letters of recommendation from elected and appointed state officials and other community leaders all assure the governor that the nominee is the person most eligible for the appointment, and blacks formerly lacked this support. A third and final consideration—and not by any means the least—was the financial sacrifice board members had to consider. On the average, board members must expect to lose fifty-to-sixty working days annually. Though members are reimbursed for travel, meals, and lodging expenses and receive a $25-to-$50 per diem allowance (amounts vary in each state) the reimbursement falls far short of the income lost while away from the office on board business. Two decades ago, this financial drain would have imposed a hardship on many black dentists and serious consideration was given before undertaking such a financially unrewarding obligation. These considerations notwithstanding, black professionals have always wanted representation on state boards and, in spite of the odds against such appointment, wished to have a voice in the regulation of dental health care and maintaining their independence and autonomy within the profession.

Notes

Introduction

1. Clifton O. Dummett, *Growth and Development of the Negro in Dentistry in the United States* (Chicago: The Stanek Press, 1952), p. 3.

Chapter II

1. The Howard University College of Dentistry, from its inception, has never drawn a color line. Until 1886 it was the only school to graduate a number of black dental professionals to meet the urgent needs of blacks. (Statistical estimates reveal that by 1885, a total of twenty-five black dentists were counted among the national total of 15,000 licensed dentists. By 1900 the total had increased to 125.)

2. Dr. Russel A. Dixon, dean emeritus of the Howard University College of Dentistry, died January 3, 1976.

Chapter III

1. American Dental Association *Journal,* February 1968, p. 233.

2. *Ibid.*

3. The address of the Student National Dental Association is P.O. Box 29, Tufts University of School of Dental Medicine, One Kneeland Street, Boston, Massachusetts, 02111.

Chapter IV

1. A list of institutions offering postgraduate or graduate courses may be obtained from the American Association of Orthodontists, 7477 Delmar Boulevard, St. Louis, Missouri 63130.

2. W. W. Bauer, Elizabeth Montgomery, and Elenore Pounds, *Health For All* (Chicago: Scott, Foresman and Company, 1966). Alexander M. Pratt, *Your Children, Their Teeth and Their Health* (Hicksville, New York: Exposition Press, 1974).

Chapter VI

1. For further information about scholarships, prospective students may write The Fund for Dental Health, 410 North Michigan Avenue, Chicago, Illinois.

Chapter VIII

1. Association for the Study of Afro-American Life and History, *International Library of Negro Life and History*, volume *The History of the Negro in Medicine* (Washington, D.C., 1970), p. 27.

Chapter X

1. *Quarterly* of the National Dental Association 28(1970): 45.

APPENDICES

Appendix A

Contributing Authors

THEODORE E. BOLDEN, D.D.S., M.S., Ph.D.
FRED BRONSON, D.D.S.
C. BASSET BROWN, D.D.S., M.S.D.
DEWITT S. DYKES, JR., B.A., M.A.
C.E. DRISKELL, D.D.S.
CLIFTON O. DUMMETT, D.D.S., M.S.D., M.P.H.
JULIANN BLUITT FOSTER, D.D.S.
HOWARD HALL, D.D.S.
NORMAN D. HALLIBURTON, C.D.T.
JOSEPH L. HENRY, D.D.S., M.S., Ph.D.
NAOMI W. LEDE, B.A., M.A., Ph.D.
WALKER MOORE, D.D.S.
LORD CECIL RHODES, D.D.S.
E. R. RICHARDSON, D.D.S., M.S.
J. B. SINGLETON, JR., D.D.S.
JEANNE SINKFORD, D.D.S., M.S., Ph.D.
BILLY WARD, D.D.S.

Advisor to the authors: DANIEL A. COLLINS, D.D.S.

Appendix B

Survey of Black Employment

Participation in

Dental Trade Establishments*

A survey was conducted during 1970 to determine the nature of the job market for black Americans in the dental industry. The study focused on the social and economic aspects of the industry as well as the attitudes of executives in industrial concerns toward hiring and promoting employees in general and black employees in particular.

The companies surveyed, selected at random from listings in *A Directory of Dental Trade Institutions,* represented a cross-section of dental trade establishments. Of the total number (158) of companies included in the initial survey, 124 returned questionnaries.

Summary of Findings

The types of dental industries included in the survey were laboratory, trade, manufacturing, mail order, pharmaceutical research, and production and marketing concerns. From the data received, 36 percent of the respondents were engaged in dental laboratories, 23 percent in trade, 36 percent in manufacturing, and approximately 5 percent in research, production, and marketing.

---

*This survey was conducted by Naomi W. Lede, director of research at Bishop College, in cooperation with the Society for the Research and Study of the Negro in Dentistry.

Total employment in all companies ranged from fifty to over one thousand, and the percentage of black employees ranged from zero to approximately 30 percent of that number, with the largest percentage of blacks employed in nonsupervisory positions.

The data also indicated that, in recent years, dental companies have begun hiring a substantial number of minority personnel. Several of the longer established companies outlined the historical origin of minority employment, and there was evidence that increasing opportunities were opening up for blacks in all areas of the industry.

Several companies indicated that blacks had been in their employ only recently. However, more than 36 percent of the companies surveyed stated that they had employed blacks for more than thirty years, although none held policy-making positions.

Table B-1
BLACK EMPLOYMENT IN DENTAL TRADE
ESTABLISHMENTS, 1970

Duration of Employment	Percentage of Blacks
6 months to 1 year	9
2 to 5 years	9
6 to 10 years	5
11 to 15 years	9
16 to 20 years	9
30 years (since company founding)	36
More than 30 years	18

Source: Naomi W. Lede, director of research, Bishop College, Dallas, Texas.
Note: Five percent of the companies surveyed did not respond.

The majority of black employees in supervisory positions were directing the activities of whites as well as other blacks. Promotional policies were considered generally the same for all employees, and salaries were commensurate with promotions and job classifications, irrespective of race, creed, or color. (None of the companies surveyed indicated that race was a major factor in hiring.) Instead, all respondents stated that their qualifications for the employment of black persons were based on competency. A few listed "Federal Contracts" as a major influence in their hiring of members of minority groups.

Employment Qualifications

Some very encouraging trends were discovered in the aggregate statistics. Despite the indication of promotions by some companies exclusively from within, and the tendency of several companies to cater to family members, the hiring of blacks for supervisory positions appeared to be somewhat more promising.

Rigid qualifications, once designed to block blacks and other disadvantaged minorities from employment, were not present in the dental occupations, according to survey data. Job qualifications appeared to be geared toward promoting better work standards for all employees and assuring high performance capabilities.

The broad conclusion of the survey, viewed within the framework of responses received, indicated that job qualifications ranged from those with no educational requirements (in some few positions), to those which required aptitude tests, college degrees, and other special requirements.

Some respondents categorized job requirements as "exempt" or "nonexempt." The exempt qualifications included having high school diplomas and/or certain other appropriate related work experience for entry-level positions; others required college degrees, as specified by the job description. The more sophisticated technical and professional positions required appropriate experience in addition to the college degree. Academic requirements for nonexempt, or "blue collar," jobs required work-related experience plus a high school school education. (Few companies stated that they required "exempt" jobs only.)

One company surveyed ran the gamut from non-high school

graduates with no related work experience to holders of the master's degrees in several fields. In this same company, job levels were varied and presented some degree of complexity, due to the fact that there were more than 800 employees, with 500 or more members of six bargaining units. A more careful examination of this company's respondents showed three job levels: exempt, nonexempt and wage. (It should be understood that within each job level were numerous classifications.

General policies for job promotions included seniority, skills, ability, dexterity, merit, attitudes, reliability, and tests. The merit promotion system employs job-bid procedure for wage employees based on performance and qualifications. The "open bidding" system, based on skill and seniority, was a common practice among the majority of the companies surveyed.

Several companies that did not respond to all items on the questionnaire indicated that there were very few black residents in their areas.

Manpower Training

Manpower training programs have been a source of recruitment for several dental trade industries. The survey indicated that on-the-job training programs placed minorities in entry-level positions with some companies. Another significant step was the participation of employers in manpower programs which focused on minority hiring and job development programs. One employer wrote, "We are participating in NABS and several OJT programs to train the disadvantaged. I personally took the AMIDS course in Washington to help me understand the minority problems better. We are interested in participating in any program . . . offered."

Another respondent, somewhat less impressed with minority hiring stated: "We work closely with the Office of Economic Opportunity (OEO) to have all minority people . . . but it is always a lost cause here . . . They just do not want to work. Minorities here are only about three percent of the population."

General Employment Information

Most of the companies surveyed indicated that employment mobility — upgrading and promotions — was the same for all employees. A large proportion of respondents chose not to answer some questions, despite provisions made to ensure anonymity. Some 68 percent of the respondents state that the employment of blacks was based on competency; 9 percent said it was not, while 23 percent gave no reply.

TABLE B-2
EMPLOYMENT POLICIES OF DENTAL TRADE ESTABLISHMENTS, 1970

Queries	Percentage of Responses		
	Yes	No	No Response
Do promotional policies apply to all employees alike?	91	9	0
Are black employees upgraded in job classification with pay commensurate with promotions?	82	0	18
Is the employment of blacks based on competency?	68	9	23
Is employment of blacks based on the race factor or quota system?	0	64	36
Is the employment of blacks based on federal contracts?	5	59	36

Source: Naomi W. Lede, director of research, Bishop College, Dallas, Texas.

A substantial number of the companies surveyed provided supplies to the offices of black dentists. In fact, 72 percent stated that they had black dentists as customers, while 9 percent said that they did not. In addition, 14 percent stated that they were not able to identify their customers by race, implying that records were not kept according to racial or ethnic origin. (This may account for the fact that 5 percent of the survey forms returned failed to respond to the question about the racial origin of their customers.)

Conclusions

Essentially, the premises upon which employment qualifications and promotions rest — as they relate to minority employment in general — are the same as those used in communicating equal employment policy. Managerial and supervisory positions are not occupied by a large number of blacks, the survey responses indicated. Whether this low percentage is due to conservative employment and promotional practices in general is difficult to assess from the data. The most frequent deterrent to the hiring of blacks for supervisory positions is the fact that promotions generally come from within rather than from outside the company, and are based on seniority.

The survey also pointed up the traditional handicaps experienced by black workers in seeking mobility in the occupational and/or corporate sturcture. Goal blockage was attributed not only to a lack of administrative experience, but the reluctance of blacks to bid for, or train for better jobs, for fear of "rocking the boat" or facing the hostility of fellow workers. In other cases, department and supervisory personnel tend to overlook blacks in their evaluation of personnel worthy of promotions. Methods of recruitment of blacks were even more inhibited by the lack of previous experience on the part of supervisors.

In developing profiles for employment policies, the majority of the companies surveyed revealed the willingness of top management to commit itself to sustained minority recruitment and hiring.

Appendix C

Black Dentists Practicing in the United States,

1930-70

State	Year				
	1930	*1940*	*1950*	*1960*	*1970*
Alabama	45	38	54	37	40
Alaska	0	0	0	1	1
Arizona	2	2	3	5	5
Arkansas	30	27	32	21	15
California	38	35	56	56	287
Colorado	4	4	2	6	6
Connecticut	13	16	24	24	31
Delaware	6	5	6	6	6
District of Columbia	72	65	90	116	157
Florida	45	39	52	54	62
Georgia	60	50	45	54	45
Hawaii	0	0	0	0	1
Idaho	0	0	0	0	0
Illinois	159	112	124	120	136
Indiana	35	32	41	38	42
Iowa	6	4	6	6	6
Kansas	14	11	14	9	8
Kentucky	37	29	27	23	20
Louisiana	45	36	40	41	46
Maine	0	0	0	0	0
Maryland	34	29	35	50	103
Massachusetts	47	30	30	35	28
Michigan	50	38	44	89	119
Minnesota	6	5	5	6	4
Mississippi	29	29	34	30	33

State	Year				
	1930	*1940*	*1950*	*1960*	*1970*
Missouri	72	47	55	50	43
Montana	0	0	0	0	0
Nebraska	7	5	3	1	2
Nevada	0	0	0	1	1
New Hampshire	0	0	0	0	0
New Jersey	73	56	76	80	100
New Mexico	2	1	1	3	4
New York	164	143	166	180	250
North Carolina	68	59	78	96	87
North Dakota	0	0	0	0	0
Ohio	96	79	63	66	58
Oklahoma	18	19	21	24	21
Oregon	1	0	0	0	0
Pennsylvania	177	131	127	167	85
Rhode Island	5	3	4	3	2
South Carolina	54	40	45	49	41
South Dakota	0	0	0	0	0
Tennessee	70	74	73	69	76
Texas	100	81	91	96	101
Utah	0	0	0	0	0
Vermont	0	0	0	0	0
Virginia	63	63	80	100	103
Washington	3	2	4	1	9
West Virginia	22	26	22	21	14
Wisconsin	6	6	8	6	8
Wyoming	0	0	0	0	0
Total	1778	1471	1681	1840	2206

Source: Figures for 1930-40 taken from Clifton O. Dummett, *Growth and Development of the Negro in Dentistry in the United States* (Chicago: The Stanek Press, 1952), pp. 77-79. Figures for 1950 taken from the *Journal* of the National Medical Association, January, 1951. Figures for 1960 compiled by Doctors Lloyd Cecil Rhodes (Norfolk, Virginia) and H. Cicero Edwards, Sr. (Washington, D.C.), cited in *Negro Handbook* edited by Ebony Editors and Doris E. Saunders (Chicago: Johnson Publishing Co., 1974), p. 324. Figures for 1970 compiled by Foster Kidd, D.D.S., and taken from his survey, 1968-70.

Appendix D

Black Dentists in Fifteen Major Metropolitan

Areas, 1967

City	Black Population	Number of Dentists
Atlanta, Georgia	186,464	22
Baltimore, Maryland	326,589	47
Birmingham, Alabama	135,113	11
Chicago, Illinois	812,637	118
Cleveland, Ohio	250,818	51
Dallas, Texas	129,242	11
Detroit, Michigan	482,223	80
Houston, Texas	215,037	40
Los Angeles, California	334,916	123
Memphis, Tennessee	184,320	24
New York, New York	1,087,931	250
Philadelphia, Pennsylvania	529,240	86
Pittsburg, Pennsylvania	100,692	25
St. Louis, Missouri	214,377	35
Washington, D.C.	411,737	157
Total	5,401,336	1,080

Source: Data collected by Foster Kidd, D.D.S., 1967.

Note: Survey taken in December 1967 of cities with a population of 100,000 or more blacks.

Appendix E

Gulf State Dental Association Survey

In January 1971, the Gulf State Dental Association's Committee on Legislation surveyed a group of Texas dentists to check their facilities, attitudes, and willingness to become involved with dental programs for the disadvantaged. Results of these findings follow:

1. General

More than two-thirds (23) of the respondents practiced dentistry in cities with populations of more than 250,000. Half of the respondents lived in areas with fluoridated water supplies. Twenty-five were in the 25-45 age group. Seventeen had been in practice for 16-25 years; seven, more than 26 years; and eight, up to 10 years. Office locations were almost equally divided between affluent downtown (16) and poverty (15) areas, but all were very accessible.

2. Patient Information

Seventy-five percent of all patients were black, and the remainder were divided almost evenly between whites and Mexican-Americans. Most of the patients surveyed visited dental offices annually. Only four dentists reported that the majority of their patients visited every six months. Extractions and fillings comprised 50-75 percent of the work load. Less than 50 percent but more than 25 percent of treatments involved crowns and bridges. Complete dentures, partials, and prosthesis accounted

119

for less than 10 percent of the work in a large number of cases.

First-time visits comprised 5 to 30 percent of their business, according to more than half of the reporting dentists. More than one-third reported 35-50 percent of their patients were seeing a dentist for the first time, and one-third reported the average age of first-time patients was younger than age ten. An almost equal number said the average was twenty-one plus. Teenagers either had been to a dentist before or were not visiting at all. Most patients seeking care for the first time had fair to very poor dental conditions.

Three-fourths of the dentists responding to the survey indicated that 57 percent of their patients were eligible for public assistance payments. An equally large number lacked dental care due to their inability to meet expenses.

3. Practice

Approximately 99 percent of all black dentists in Texas are in solo practice with two or more operatories. All dentists surveyed had convenient office hours (9 a.m. to 6 p.m.), offered emergency hours, and were seeking an average of 100 patients weekly. All of the dentists employed one to three auxiliary personnel; most would employ another dentist if one were available. Almost 90 percent of the dentists treated children or had adequate referral outlets. More than one-third of these dentists would treat children as early as age three.

4. Federal or State and Local Programs

The dentists surveyed felt present programs in their state did not adequately meet the needs of the target population. They favored: 1. dental inclusion in National Health Insurance Programs; 2. the private office setting for treatment; 3. Medicaid in Texas, including dental services; and 4. AFDC Programs (Aid to Dependent Children) to provide additional dental services, too.

These data, if generalized to include all of the dentists in Texas and projected to include other states, also, show that black and minority dentists are concerned about the disadvantaged and are willing to foster programs to provide adequate dental care for those on welfare. The shortage of dentists previously referred to is based on actual numerical count. Hence, these data are not to be construed to mean that every dental office is overloaded with patients and that all dentists are overworked; the demand has not yet equaled the need for services, hence figures showing dentist-to-population ratios are more useful if viewed academically.

Appendix F

Black Dental Student Population, 1975-76

State	Dental School	Total Students	Total Blacks	Total in State
Alabama	University of Alabama	266	12	12
California	University of the Pacific	404	1	
	University of California at Los Angeles	421	24	
	University of Southern California	519	26	
	Loma Linda University	291	8	
	University of California at San Francisco	352	24	83
Colorado	University of Colorado	73		
Connecticut	University of Connecticut	159	5	5
District of Columbia	Georgetown University	579	12	
	Howard University	396	302	314
Florida	University of Florida	147	6	6
Georgia	Emory University	411	1	
	Medical College of Georgia	180	20	21
Illinois	Loyola University	536	7	
	Northwestern University	406	1	
	University of Illinois	530	19	
	Southern Illinois University	124	1	28
Indiana	Indiana University	508	6	6
Iowa	University of Iowa	359	6	6

State	Dental School	Total Students	Total Blacks	Total in State
Kentucky	University of Kentucky	247	12	
	University of Louisville	334	3	15
Louisiana	Louisiana State University	374	4	4
Maryland	University of Maryland	521	35	35
Massachusetts	Harvard University	79	9	
	Tufts University	438	18	
	Boston University	103	1	28
Michigan	University of Detroit	286	15	
	University of Michigan	593	46	61
Minnesota	University of Minnesota	565	5	5
Mississippi	University of Mississippi	25	2	2
Missouri	University of Missouri at Kansas City	632	10	
	Washington University	289	6	16
Nebraska	The Creighton University	287	14	
	University of Nebraska	257	0	14
New Jersey	Fairleigh Dickinson University	325	10	
	New Jersey College of Dentistry	195	16	26
New York	Columbia University	206	3	
	New York University	584	10	
	State University of New York at Buffalo	353	13	
	State University of New York at Stony Brook	69	4	30
North Carolina	University of North Carolina	329	10	10
Ohio	Ohio State University	748	8	
	Case Western Reserve University	396	13	21
Oklahoma	University of Oklahoma	107	5	5
Oregon	University of Oregon	316	5	5
Pennsylvania	Temple University	573	11	
	University of Pennsylvania	634	13	
	University of Pittsburg	528	22	46

State	Dental School	Total Students	Total Blacks	Total in State
South Carolina	Medical University of South Carolina	165	6	6
Tennessee	Meharry Medical College	158	131	
	University of Tennessee	467	7	138
Texas	Baylor University	368	4	
	University of Texas at Houston	491	6	
	University of Texas at San Antonio	245	2	12
Virginia	Virginia Commonwealth University	442	10	10
Washington	University of Washington	378	5	5
West Virginia	West Virginia University	241	2	2
Wisconsin	Marquette University	540	0	0
Puerto Rico	University of Puerto Rico	218	0	0
Total		20,767	977	977

Source: Minority Report, Dental Education Supplement No. 3, compiled from *The Annual Survey of Dental Educational Institutions,* Division of Educational Measurements, American Dental Association (Chicago, Illinois, 1976).

Appendix G

Dental School Admission Requirements

and Accredited Dental Schools

Dental School admission committees will consider the applications of candidates who present the following minimal qualifications:

1. Graduation from an approved secondary school, or the equivalent in entrance examinations.

2. At least two full academic years of acceptable college credit earned in a college or Institute of Technology, currently approved by an agency recognized by the Council on Dental Education of the American Dental Association.

These agencies are:

- a. Middle States Association of Colleges and Secondary Schools.
- b. New England Association of Colleges and Secondary Schools.
- c. North Central Association of Colleges and Secondary Schools.
- d. Northwest Association of Secondary and Higher Schools.
- e. Southern Association of Colleges and Schools.
- f. Western Association of Schools and Colleges.

3. The satisfactory completion of the two years pre-education by September of the year the applicant desires to be admitted, with the following courses and credits indicated:

	Semester Hours	Quarter Hours
a. Biology or Zoology	8	12
b. Inorganic Chemistry	8	12
c. Organic Chemistry	8	12
d. Physics	8	12
e. English Composition	6	9

Comparative Anatomy and Embryology are strongly recommended. It is also highly recommended that the applicant supplement these basic requirements with courses in the humanities, social sciences, and other elective courses, such as: mechanical drawing, mathematics, economics, history, psychology, foreign languages, philosophy, fine arts, and logic.

The high school graduate aspiring to any of the healing arts professions should be sure that the college or university of his choice offers these necessary prerequisites.

The procedure for applying is generally similar, but may vary slightly from college to college. The applicant should follow the course set fourth by the school(s) of his choice. For detailed information on procedures for admission, write to the Registrar, or dean of the dental schools on the following list.

There are 59 dental schools in the United States, 35 of which are classified as public institutions and 24 as private:

ALABAMA

School of Dentistry, University of Alabama
University Station
Birmingham, 35294
Dean: Dr. Charles A. McCallum, Jr.

CALIFORNIA

School of Dentistry, Loma Linda University
Loma Linda, 92354
Dean: Dr. Judson Klooster

School of Dentistry, University of California at Los Angeles
Center for the Health Sciences
Los Angeles, 90024
Dean: Dr. Andrew D. Dixon

School of Dentistry, University of California
San Francisco, 94143
Dean: Dr. Ben W. Pavone

School of Dentistry, University of the Pacific
2155 Webster Street
San Francisco, 94115
Dean: Dr. Dale F. Redig

School of Dentistry, University of Southern California
925 W. 34th Street
Los Angeles, 90007
Dean: Dr. William H. Crawford

CONNECTICUT

School of Dental Medicine, The University of Connecticut
263 Farmington Avenue
Farmington, 06032
Dean: Dr. Harald Löe

DISTRICT OF COLUMBIA

School of Dentistry, Georgetown University
3900 Reservoir Road, N.W.
Washington, D.C. 20007
Dean: Dr. Charles B. Murto

College of Dentistry, Howard University
600 W Street, N.W.
Washington, D.C. 20059
Dean: Dr. Jeanne C. Sinkford

GEORGIA

School of Dentistry, Emory University
1462 Clifton Road, N.E.
Atlanta, 30322
Dean: Dr. George H. Moulton

School of Dentistry, Medical College of Georgia
1459 Gwinnett Street
Augusta, 30902
Dean: Dr. Judson C. Hickey

ILLINOIS

College of Dentistry, University of Illinois
801 S. Paulina Street
Chicago, 60612
Dean: Dr. Seymour H. Yale

Northwestern University Dental School
311 E. Chicago Avenue
Chicago, 60611
Dean: Dr. Norman H. Olsen

School of Dentistry, Loyola University
2160 S. First Avenue
Maywood, 60153
Dean: Dr. Raffaele Suriano

School of Dental Medicine
Southern Illinois University
Edwardsville, 62025
Dean: Dr. Vasil Vasileff (Acting)

INDIANA

School of Dentistry, Indiana University
1121 W. Michigan Street
Indianapolis, 46202
Dean: Dr. Ralph E. McDonald

IOWA

College of Dentistry, The University of Iowa
Dental Building
Iowa City, 52242
Dean: Dr. Richard Miller

KENTUCKY

College of Dentistry, University of Kentucky
800 Rose Street
Lexington, 40506
Dean: Dr. Merrill W. Packer

School of Dentistry, University of Louisville
Health Sciences Center
Louisville, 40201
Dean: Dr. Merwyn A. Landay

LOUISIANA

School of Dentistry, Louisiana State University
1100 Florida Avenue
New Orleans, 70119
Dean: Dr. Edmund E. Jeansonne

MARYLAND

Baltimore College of Dental Surgery
Dental School, University of Maryland
666 West Baltimore Street
Baltimore, 21201
Dean: Dr. Errol L. Reese

MASSACHUSETTS

Harvard School of Dental Medicine
188 Longwood Avenue
Boston, 02115
Dean: Dr. Paul Goldhaber

School of Dental Medicine, Tufts University
One Kneeland Street
Boston, 02111
Dean: Dr. Robert B. Shira

School of Graduate Dentistry, Boston University
100 E. Newton Street
Boston, 02118
Dean: Dr. Henry M. Goldman

MICHIGAN

School of Dentistry, The University of Michigan
Ann Arbor, 48104
Dean: Dr. William R. Mann

School of Dentistry, University of Detroit
2985 E. Jefferson Avenue
Detroit, 48297
Acting Dean: Dr. Daniel Goodman

MINNESOTA

School of Dentistry, University of Minnesota
515 Delaware Street, S.E.
Minneapolis, 55455
Dean: Dr. Richard C. Oliver

MISSOURI

School of Dentistry, University of Missouri at Kansas City
650 E. 25th Street
Kansas City, 64108
Dean: Dr. Marvin E. Revzin

School of Dental Medicine, Washington University
4559 Scott Avenue
St. Louis, 63110
Dean: Dr. John T. Bird, Jr.

NEBRASKA

College of Dentistry, University of Nebraska
40th and Holdredge Streets
Lincoln, 68503
Dean: Dr. Richard E. Bradley

Boyne School of Dental Science, Creighton University
2500 California Street
Omaha, 68178
Dean: Dr. Robert V. Vining

NEW JERSEY

New Jersey Dental School
100 Bergen Street
Newark, 07103
Dean: Dr. Theodore E. Bolden

School of Dentistry, Fairleigh Dickinson University
110 Fuller Place
Hacken Sack, 07601
Dean: Dr. Ralph S. Kaslick

NEW YORK

School of Dentistry, State University of New York at Buffalo
3435 Main Street
Buffalo, 14214
Dean: Dr. William M. Feagans

School of Dentistry and Oral Surgery, Columbia University
630 W. 168th Street
New York, 10032
Dean: Dr. Edward V. Legarelli

College of Dentistry, New York University
Brookdale Dental Center, 421 First Avenue
New York, 10010
Dean: Dr. Donald B. Giddon

School of Dental Medicine
State University of New York
Stony Brook 11790
Dean: Dr. Leo M. Sneelny

NORTH CAROLINA

School of Dentistry, University of North Carolina
Chapel Hill, 27514
Dean: Dr. Raymond P. White

OHIO

School of Dentistry, Case-Western Reserve University
2123 Abington Road
Cleveland, 44106
Acting Dean: Dr. Thomas J. DeMarco

College of Dentistry, Ohio State University
305 W. 12th Avenue
Columbus, 43210
Dean: Dr. Charles L. Howell

OREGON

University of Oregon Dental School
611 SW Campus Dr.
Portland, 97201
Dean: Dr. Louis G. Terkla

PENNSYLVANIA

School of Dental Medicine, University of Pennsylvania
4001 W. Spruce Street
Philadelphia, 19104
Dean: Dr. D. Walter Cohen

School of Dentistry, Temple University
3223 N. Broad Street
Philadelphia, 19122
Acting Dean: Dr. Dale F. Roeck

School of Dental Medicine, University of Pittsburgh
3501 Terrace Street
Pittsburgh, 15261
Dean: Dr. Edward J. Forrest

PUERTO RICO

School of Dentistry, University of Puerto Rico
GPO Box 5067
San Juan, 00936
Dean: Dr. Carlos L. Suárez

SOUTH CAROLINA

College of Dental Medicine, Medical University of South Carolina
80 Barre Street
Charleston, 29401
Acting Dean: Dr. Arthur L. Haisten

TENNESSEE

College of Dentistry, University of Tennessee
847 Monroe Avenue
Memphis, 38163
Dean: Dr. Jack E. Wells

School of Dentistry, Meharry Medical College
1005 18th Avenue, N.
Nashville, 37208
Dean: Dr. Eugenia Mobley

TEXAS

The University of Texas, Health Sciences at Houston
Dental Branch
PO Box 20068
Houston, 77025
Dean: Dr. John V. Olson

Baylor College of Dentistry
800 Hall Street
Dallas, 75226
Dean: Dr. Kenneth V. Randolph

The University of Texas, Dental School of San Antonio
7703 Floyd Curl Drive
San Antonio, 78284
Dean: Dr. Philip J. Boyne

VIRGINIA

School of Dentistry, Virginia Commonwealth University
520 N. 12th Street
Richmond, 23298
Dean: Dr. John A. DiBiaggio

WASHINGTON

School of Dentistry, University of Washington
Health Sciences Building
Seattle, 98105
Dean: Dr. Alton W. Moore

WEST VIRGINIA

School of Dentistry, West Virginia University
The Medical Center
Morgantown, 26506
Dean: Dr. W. Robert Biddington

WISCONSIN

School of Dentistry, Marquette University
604 N. 16th Street
Milwaukee, 53233
Dean: Dr. Russell V. Brown

New Programs Not Fully Operational

COLORADO

School of Dentistry, University of Colorado
Medical Center
4200 E. 9th Avenue
Denver, 80220
Dean: Dr. Leslie R. Burrows
(First-year class enrolled in 1973)

FLORIDA

College of Dentistry, University of Florida
J. Hillis Miller Health Center
Gainesville, 32601
Dean: Dr. Don L. Allen
(First-year class enrolled in 1972)

MISSISSIPPI

School of Dentistry, University of Mississippi
2500 N. State Street
Jackson, 39216
Dean: Dr. Wallace V. Mann, Jr.
(First-year class enrolled in 1975)

NEW YORK

School of Dental Medicine, State University of New York at Stony Brook
Stony Brook, 11794
Dean: Dr. Leo M. Sreebny
(First-year class enrolled in 1973)

OKLAHOMA

College of Dentistry, The University of Oklahoma
1110 N. E. 12th Street
PO Box 26901
Oklahoma City, 73190
Dean: Dr. William E. Brown
(First-year class enrolled in 1972)

CANADA

Reciprocal agreement between the Council on Education of the Canadian
Dental Association and the Council on Dental Education of the American
Dental Association to recognize programs as accredited.

Faculty of Dentistry, University of Alberta
3036 Dental-Pharmacy Centre
Edmonton, Alberta, T6G-2N8
Dean: Dr. James McCutcheon

Faculty of Dentistry, University of British Columbia
2075 Westbrook Place
Vancouver, British Columbia, V6T-1W5
Dean: Dr. S. Wah Leung

Faculty of Dentistry, Dalhousie University
Dentistry Building
5981 University Avenue
Halifax, Nova Scotia, B3H-3J5
Acting Dean: Dr. Robert H. Bingham

Ecole de Médecine Dentaire, Université Laval
Québec, G1K-7P4
Dean: Dr. Paul Simard

Faculty of Dentistry, University of Manitoba
780 Bannatyne Avenue
Winnipeg, Manitoba, R3E-0W3
Dean: Dr. John W. Neilson

Faculty of Dentistry, McGill University
PO Box 6070, Station A
Montreal, Quebec, H3C-3G1
Dean: Dr. E. R. Ambrose

Faculté de Médecine Dentaire
Université de Montréal
CP 6209, Succursale A
Montreal, Quebec, H3C-3J7
Dean: Dr. Jean-Paul Lussier

College of Dentistry, University of Saskatchewan
Saskatoon, Saskatchewan, S7N-0W0
Dean: Dr. C. W. B. McPhail

Faculty of Dentistry, University of Toronto
124 Edward Street
Toronto, Ontario, M5G-1G6
Dean: Dr. Gordon Nikiforuk

Faculty of Dentistry, University of Western Ontario
1151 Richmond Street
London, Ontario, N6A-5B7
Dean: Dr. Wesley J. Dunn

For information about accredited dental hygiene, dental assisting, and dental laboratory technology programs, write:

American Dental Association
Commission on Accreditation
211 E. Chicago Avenue
Chicago, Illinois 60611

Appendix H

Scholarship and Loan Sources

American Fund for Dental Health

The American Fund for Dental Health was created in 1955 as the national agency for collection and distribution of voluntary contributions to support dental education. The fund is sponsored by the American Dental Association, the American Association of Dental Schools, and the American Dental Trade Association. Interest loans are available to students at each dental school from the ADA-AFDE Student Loan Fund. The American Dental Association contributes financially to the program through the American Fund for Dental Health which distributes the funds to dental schools. The loans are administered by each school in accordance with its student aid policies. Information on the availability and repayment provisions of the loans should be obtained from the school of the student's choice.

American Dental Trade Association — Student Loan Fund

Junior and senior dental students in the United States and Canada may be recommended by the dean of the dental school to receive American Dental Trade Association student loans. (An amount up to $700 may be borrowed.) The loan is repayable within two years from the date of graduation at an interest rate of 3 percent per annum. Additional information concerning ADTA loans may be obtained from the individual dental schools.

International College of Dentists (U.S.A. Section)

Dental schools in the United States receive grants from the International College of Dentists' Student Loan Fund to provide financial assistance to senior students. Dental schools administer the fund and determine qualifications and other provisions according to their customary loan policies. Additional information may be obtained from any dental school.

W. K. Kellogg Foundation

The W. K. Kellogg Foundation has provided grants to dental schools in the United States and Canada for the establishment of undergraduate student loan funds since 1941. Funds are administered by each school in accordance with its student aid policies and are restricted to undergraduate dental students at low interest rates. Each dental school can provide additional information on qualifications, loan limitations, and repayment provisions.

Southern Regional Education Board

Students who are residents of Alabama, Arkansas, Florida, Louisiana, Maryland, Mississippi, North Carolina, Oklahoma, South Carolina, Tennessee, Texas, and Virginia may apply for aid from the Southern Regional Education Board Regional Contract Program. Participating states pay a supplementary fee, thereby reducing the tuition cost to the student. For additional information write to: Southern Regional Education Board, 130 Sixth Street, NW, Atlanta, Georgia 30313.

Smith-Holden Scholarships

Four $300 scholarships are provided each year to residents of Connecticut, Rhode Island, Massachusetts, and New Hampshire. Scholarships are administered by the state dental societies of the four states, and eligibility is determined by the society. For additional information write to: Smith-Holden Inc., 99 Corliss Street, Providence, Rhode Island.

U.S. Government-Health Professions Education Assistance Act

The Congress of the United States enacted the Health Professions Education Assistance Act in 1963. A provision of the Act established federal loans for students of dentistry. Eligible students may borrow up to $2,500 per year during each year of their undergraduate professional education. Preference is given to freshmen dental students who would not otherwise be able to finance dental education. Loans carry low interest rates and must be repaid within ten years, commencing three years after the recipient graduates or leaves school.

In 1965, the Congress amended the Health Professions Education Assistance Act to provide scholarship funds for dental students. Each dental school in the United States now receives funds for scholarship support of a limited number of dental students. Fund reference is again given to the prospective freshman student who could not enter a dental school without financial support and whose financial situation does not qualify him for a low interest loan. The scholarships are awarded in amounts up to $2,500 per year and are administered by the schools. Additional information on the federal scholarship and loan programs can be obtained from the dental schools.

Western Interstate Commission for Higher Education

Dental students who are residents of Alaska, Arizona, California, Hawaii, Idaho, Montana, Nevada, New Mexico, and Wyoming may apply for aid under the Western Interstate Commission for Higher Education program. These states pay participating dental schools a supplementary fee, thereby lowering the tuition cost to the student. Participating dental schools are: College of Physicians and Surgeons, Loma Linda University, University of California at Los Angeles, University of California at San Francisco, University of Southern California, University of Oregon, and the University of Washington. Further information is available from the Western Interstate Commission for Higher Education, University East Campus, 30th Street, Boulder, Colorado 80304.

United Student Aid Funds

United Student Aid Funds is a private, nonprofit corporation which endorses low cost loans made by the student's hometown financial institution. Undergraduates may borrow up to $1,000 per year, graduate students may borrow up to $1,500 per year, or a combined total of not more than $7,500. Repayment of loans begins on the first day of the tenth month after the student leaves school. Monthly installments usually are not less than $25 nor more than $100. Additional information relative to USA Funds loans may be obtained from the financial officer of any accredited school.

Other Dental School Loans

Many dental schools have at their disposal limited funds for financial aid to dental students. Information about these funds should be obtained from the individual schools. Generally, funds are made available to students on the basis of academic achievement and need.

Dental Auxiliaries

Schools offering an educational program in one of the dental auxiliaries (dental hygiene, dental assisting, or dental laboratory technology) have at their disposal funds for the provision of financial aid to dental auxiliary students. Information about these funds should be obtained from the individual schools.

In addition, limited scholarships and loans are available through the following organizations:

American Dental Assistants Association
211 E Chicago Avenue
Chicago, Illinois 60611

(For Dental Laboratory Technology Scholarships)
American Fund for Dental Health
211 E Chicago Avenue
Chicago, Illinois 60611

American Dental Hygienists Association
211 E. Chicago Avenue
Chicago, Illinois 60611

Other Financial Aid Sources

The following list represents funds reported by constituent and component dental societies. Inquiries regarding a particular fund should be directed to the society at the address shown.

ARIZONA

Arizona State Dental Association
Student Loan Fund
3800 N. Central Avenue
Phoenix, Arizona 85012

DELAWARE

Delaware Academy of Medicine, Inc.
Scholarship Loan Fund
1925 Lovering Avenue
Wilmington Delaware 19806

FLORIDA

Florida State Dental Society
Student Loan Fund
P.O. Box 1810
Tampa, Florida 33609

INDIANA

Indiana State Dental Association
Student Loan Fund Program
721 Hume Mansur Building
Indianapolis, Indiana 46204

IOWA

University of Iowa
Achievement Fund
Iowa Memorial Union
Iowa City, Iowa 52240

IDA Student Loan Fund
University of Iowa Foundation
Iowa Memorial Union
Iowa City, Iowa 52240

KANSAS

Kansas State Dental Auxiliary Loan Fund
School of Dentistry
University of Missouri at Kansas City
Kansas City, Missouri

KENTUCKY

Memorial Student Loan Fund
Kentucky Dental Association
1940 Princeton Drive
Louisville, Kentucky 40205

Kentucky State Board of Dental Examiners Rural Scholarship
(Kentucky Dental)
2106 Bardstown Road
Louisville, Kentucky 40205

LOUISIANA

Women's Auxiliary to the Louisiana Dental Association
Dental Student Loan Fund
10 Stilt Street
New Orleans, Louisiana 70124

MAINE

Maine Dental Association
Student Loan Fund
Bethel, Maine 04217

MASSACHUSETTS

Massachusetts Dental Society
Dental Student Financial Aid Committee
The Prudential Tower Building
Suite 4318
Boston, Massachusetts 02199

South Shore District Dental Society Loan Fund
47 W. Elm Street
Brockton, Massachusetts 02401

MINNESOTA

Minnesota State Dental Association Student Loan Fund
2236 Marshall Avenue
St. Paul, Minnesota 55104

Information regarding the following loans can be obtained from: School of Dentistry, University of Minnesota, Washington Avenue and Union Street, S.E. Minneapolis, Minnesota 55455:

Duluth District Auxiliary Loan Fund
Minneapolis District Auxiliary Loan Fund
Northwestern District Auxiliary Loan Fund
Saint Paul District Auxiliary Loan Fund
Southeastern District Loan Fund

NEBRASKA

The Dr. Clyde W. Davis Student Loan Fund
University of Nebraska
Office of Scholarships and Financial Aids
Administration Building 205
Lincoln, Nebraska 68508

NEVADA

Nevada State Dental Society Loan Fund
P.O. Box 646
Sparks, Nevada 89431

NEW HAMPSHIRE

Walter F. Winchester and New Hampshire Dental Society Memorials
Scholarship Fund
Chairman, Scholarship Fund Committee
19 Temple Court
Manchester, New Hampshire 03104

MacRury Scholarship Find for Dental Hygiene Students
188 Cody Street
Manchester, New Hampshire 03103

NEW JERSEY

Scholarship and Loan Committee
Bergen County Dental Society
Englewood, New Jersey 07631

NEW MEXICO

New Mexico Dental Association
Student Loan Fund
2917 Santa Cruz Avenue, S.E.
Albuquerque, New Mexico 87106

NORTH CAROLINA

North Carolina Dental Society
Dental Student Loan Fund
P.O. Box 11065
Raleigh, North Carolina 27604

SOUTH CAROLINA

South Carolina Dental Association
Student Loan
1506 Gregg Street
Columbia, South Carolina 29201

TENNESSEE

L. G. Noel Memorial Foundation
Student Loan Fund
307 East F Street
Elizabethton, Tennessee 37643

VERMONT

Dr. C. I. Taggart Memorial Fund
University of Vermont
590 Main Street
Burlington, Vermont 05401

VIRGINIA

Virginia State Dental Association
Student Loan Fund
Medical College of Virginia, School of Dentistry
521 N. 11th Street
Richmond, Virginia 23219

Dental Hygienists Scholarship Loan Funds
Virginia State Loan Association
18 N. Fifth Street
Richmond, Virginia 23219

WASHINGTON

Womens Auxiliary
Washington Dental Association
Student Scholarship Fund (State)
417 Grosvenor House
500 Wall Street
Seattle, Washington 98121

WEST VIRGINIA

Auxiliary of the West Virginia State Dental Society,
Dental School Loan Fund
School of Dentistry
West Virginia University
The Medical Center
Morgantown, West Virginia 26506

WISCONSIN
Wisconsin Dental Association Foundation
Student Loan Fund
633 W. Wisconsin Avenue
Milwaukee, Wisconsin 53203

Appendix I

Accredited Advanced Training Programs

in Oral Surgery

Name and Location of Program	Length of Program (years)	Annual Openings
AIR FORCE		
David Grant USAF Hospital Travis AFB, California 94535	2	1
Wilford Hall USAF Hospital Lackland Air Force Base San Antonio, Texas 78236	3	1
ARMY		
Letterman General Hospital Presidio of San Francisco, California 94129	3	1
Fitzsimmons General Hospital Denver, Colorado 80240	3	1
Walter Reed Army Medical Hospital Center, Washington, D.C. 20012	2	1
U.S. Army Tripler Hospital Honolulu, Hawaii 96819	2	1
Womack Army Hospital Fort Bragg, North Carolina 28307	2	1
William Beaumont General Hospital El Paso, Texas 79920	2	1

Name and Location of Program	Length of Program (years)	Annual Openings
Brooke General Hospital Brooke Army Medical Center Fort Sam Houston San Antonio, Texas 78234	2	1
Madigan General Hospital Tacoma, Washington 98431	2	1
VETERANS ADMINISTRATION		
Veterans Administration Hospital 700 S. 19th Street Birmingham, Alabama 35233	3	1
Veterans Administration Hospital 5901 E. 7th Street Long Beach, California 90801	3	1
Veterans Administration Hospital Washington, D.C. 20422	1	1
Veterans Administration Hospital 1670 Clairmont Road, N.E. Atlanta, Georgia 30329	2	1
Veterans Administration Hospital Hines, Illinois 60141	2	1
Veterans Administration Hospital Wadsworth, Kansas	3	1
Veterans Administration Hospital Boston, Massachusetts 02132	3	1
Veterans Administration Hospital Allen Park, Michigan 48101	3	1
Veterans Administration Hospital 4801 Linwood Boulevard Kansas City, Missouri 64128	3	1
Veterans Administration Hospital East Orange, New Jersey 07019	2	1

Name and Location of Program	Length of Program (years)	Annual Openings
Veterans Adminstration Hospital 130 West Kingsbridge Road Bronx, New York 10468	3	1
Veterans Administration Hospital Brooklyn, New York 11209	2	1
Veterans Administration Hospital 3495 Bailey Avenue Buffalo, New York 14215	3	1
Veterans Administration Hospital Fulton Street and Erwin Road Durham, North Carolina 27705	3	1
Veterans Administration Hospital Philadelphia, Pennsylvania 19104	1	1
Veterans Administration Hospital University Drive Pittsburgh, Pennsylvania 15240	3	1
Veterans Administration Hospital 2002 Holcombe Boulevard Houston, Texas 77031	3	1
Veterans Administration Hospital Wood, Wisconsin 53193	3	
CALIFORNIA		
Advanced Training Program in Oral Surgery Loma Linda University Loma Linda, 92354	3	1-2
Advanced Training Program in Oral Surgery UCLA Hospital Medical Center Los Angeles, 90024	3	1
University of Southern California 925 34th Street Los Angeles, 90007	3	3

Name and Location of Program	Length of Program (years)	Annual Openings
Highland-Alameda County Hospital 2701-14th Avenue Oakland, 94006	3-4	2
San Francisco Hospital University of California Service 22nd and Potrero Streets San Francisco, 94110	1	2
San Francisco Medical Center San Francisco, 94122	3	2
COLORADO		
Denver General Hospital W. 6th at Cherokee Street Denver, 80204	2	1
CONNECTICUT		
Hartford Hospital 80 Seymour Street Hartford, 06115	2	1
St. Francis Hospital 114 Woodland Street Hartford, 06105	2	1
Hospital of St. Raphael 1450 Chapel Street New Haven, 06510	3	1
DELAWARE		
The Wilmington Medical Center Washington and 14th Streets Wilmington, 19899	2	2
DISTRICT OF COLUMBIA		
Howard University 600 W. Street N.W. Washington, 20009	3	3

Name and Location of Program	Length of Program (years)	Annual Openings
Georgetown University 3900 Reservoir Road Washington, 20007	3	4
Washington Hospital Center 110 Irving Street, N.W. Washington, 20010	3	2
FLORIDA		
Duval Medical Center 2000 Jefferson Street Jacksonville, 32206	2	1
Jackson Memorial Hospital 1700 N. 10th Avenue Miami, 33136	2	2
GEORGIA		
Grady Memorial Hospital 80 Butler Street Atlanta, 30303	2	2
Medical College of Georgia Augusta, 30902	3	2
ILLINOIS		
Cook County Hospital 1825 W. Harrison Street Chicago, 60612	2	3
Franklin Boulevard Hospital 3240 W. Franklin Street Chicago, 60624	2	1
Loyola University of Chicago 2160 S. First Avenue Maywood, 60153	1	6
Michael Reese Hospital and Medical Center 2929 S. Ellis Chicago, 60616	3	1

Name and Location of Program	Length of Program (years)	Annual Openings
Northwestern University Dental School 311 E. Chicago Avenue Chicago, 60611	3	1
University of Illinois P.O. Box 6998 Chicago, 60608	3	3
University of Chicago Hospitals and Clinics Zoller Memorial Dental Clinic 950 E. 59th Street Chicago, 60637	3	1
Carle Memorial Hospital 602 W. University Avenue Urbana, 61801	2	1
INDIANA		
Indiana University Medical Center 1100 W. Michigan Avenue Indianapolis, 46202	3	2
Marion County General Hospital 960 Locke Street Indianapolis, 46202	3	2
IOWA		
University of Iowa University Hospitals Iowa City, 52240	3	3
KENTUCKY		
University of Kentucky A.B. Chandler Medical Center Lexington, 40506	3	2
University of Louisville Hospitals 323 E. Chestnut Street Louisville, 40202	3	2

Name and Location of Program	Length of Program (years)	Annual Openings
LOUISIANA		
Charity Hospital of Louisiana at New Orleans 1532 Tulane Avenue New Orleans, 70140	3	5
Ochsner Foundation Hospital 1516 Jefferson Highway New Orleans, 70121	3	1
Confederate Memorial Medical Center 1541 Kings Highway Shreveport, 71101	3	2
MARYLAND		
Mercy Hospital, Inc. Calvert and Saratoga Streets Baltimore, 21202	1	1
Johns Hopkins Hospital 601 N. Broadway Baltimore, 21205	3	2
University of Maryland Hospital Redwood and Green Streets Baltimore, 21201	3-4	3
MASSACHUSETTS		
Boston University 80 E. Concord Boston, 02118	1	15
Massachusetts General Hospital Fruit Street Boston, 02114	3	2
Tufts University 136 Harrison Avenue Boston, 02155	3	5

Name and Location of Program	Length of Program (years)	Annual Openings
MICHIGAN		
The University of Michigan Ann Arbor, 48104	3	3
Detroit General Hospital 1326 St. Antonine Street Detroit, 48226	3	1
Henry Ford Hospital 2799 W. Grand Boulevard Detroit, 48202	3	2
Sinai Hospital of Detroit 6767 W. Outer Drive Detroit, 48235	3	1
MINNESOTA		
University of Minnesota Washington Avenue and Union Street, S.E. Minneapolis, 55455	3	3
Mayo Graduate School of Medicine 200 First Street, W. Rochester, 55901	3	4
MISSOURI		
University of Missouri at Kansas City 1108 E. 10th Street Kansas City, 64106	3	3
Washington University 4559 Scott Avenue St. Louis, 63110	1	2
NEBRASKA		
The University of Nebraska Medical Center 42nd Street and Dewey Avenue Omaha, 68105	3	2

Name and Location of Program	Length of Program (years)	Annual Openings
NEW JERSEY		
New Jersey Medical Center 50 Baldwin Avenue Jersey City, 07304	2	2
Martlend Hospital Unit New Jersey College of Medicine and Dentistry 65 Bergen Street Newark, 07170	1	1
NEW YORK		
Bronx Municipal Hospital Center Pelham Parkway and Eastchester Road Bronx, 10461	3	2
Lincoln Hospital 333 Southern Boulevard Bronx, 10454	3	3
Misericordia-Fordham Hospital Southern Boulevard and Crotona Avenue Bronx, 10458	3	2
Morrisania City Hospital 166th Street and Gerard Avenue Bronx, 10452	1	1
Cumberland Hospital 39 Auburn Place Brooklyn, 11205	3	3
Jewish Hospital and Medical Center of Brooklyn 300 S. Skillman Brooklyn, 11211	3	3
Kings County Hospital Center 451 Clarkson Avenue Brooklyn, 11203	2	5
Coney Island Hospital 2601 Ocean Parkway Brooklyn, 11235	2	4

Name and Location of Program	Length of Program (years)	Annual Openings
Buffalo General Hospital 100 High Street Buffalo, 14203	3	1
Millard Fillmore Hospital 3 Gates Circle Buffalo, 14209	3	1
State University of New York at Buffalo Capen Hall, 15 The Circle Buffalo, 14214	3	1
City Hospital Center at Elmhurst 79-01 Broadway Elmhurst, 11373	3	4
Long Island Jewish Hospital Queens Hospital Center Affiliation 82-68 164th Street Jamaica, 11432	2	3
Columbia University 630 W. 168th New York, 10032	2	6
Metropolitan Hospital 1901 First Avenue New York, 10029	2	2
The Mount Sinai Hospital 11 E. 100th Street New York, 10029	3	4
The New York Hospital 525 E. 68th Street New York, 10021	2	1
New York University 421 First Avenue New York, 10010	3	6
Roosevelt Hospital 428 W. 59th Street New York, 10019	2	1

Name and Location of Program	Length of Program (years)	Annual Openings
St. Luke's Hospital Center Amsterdam Avenue and 114th Street Morningside Heights New York, 10025	3	1
University of Rochester School of Medicine and Dentistry 260 Crittenden Street Rochester, 14620	3	5
Grasslands Hospital Valhalla, 10595	2	1
NORTH CAROLINA		
Duke University Medical Center Durham, 27706	3	1
OHIO		
Cincinnati General Hospital 3231 Burnet Avenue Cincinnati, 45229	3	2
Cleveland Metropolitan General Hospital 3395 Scranton Road Cleveland, 44109	2	2
Case-Western Reserve University 2165 Adelbert Road Cleveland, 44106	3	1
University Hospital 410 W. 10th Avenue Columbus, 43210	3	3
St. Elizabeth Hospital 1044 Belmont Avenue Youngstown, 44505	1	1

Name and Location of Program	Length of Program (years)	Annual Openings
OKLAHOMA		
Oklahoma University Medical Center 800 N.E. 13th Street Oklahoma City, 73104	3	3
PENNSYLVANIA		
Geisinger Medical Center Danville, 17821	2	1
Harrisburg Hospital 1711 N. Front Street Harrisburg, 17102	2	1
Episcopal Hospital Front and Lehigh Avenue Philadelphia, 19125	2	1
Advanced Training Program in Oral Surgery Hahnemann Medical College and Hospital Philadelphia, 19102	3	1
Jefferson Medical College Hospital 11th and Walnut Streets Philadelphia, 19107	2	1-2
Pennsylvania Hospital 8th and Spruce Streets Philadelphia, 19107	2	2
Philadelphia General Hospital Blockley Division 34th Street and Curie Avenue Philadelphia, 19104	3	1
Presbyterian University of Pennsylvania Medical Center 51 N. 39th Street Philadelphia, 19194	1	2
Temple University 3223 N. Broad Street Philadelphia, 19122	3	1

Name and Location of Program	Length of Program (years)	Annual Openings
University of Pennsylvania 4001 Spruce Street Philadelphia, 19104	3	2
Allegheny General Hospital 320 E. North Avenue Pittsburgh, 15212	3	1
Magee Woman's Hospital Forges Avenue and Halket Street Pittsburgh, 15213	1	1
Montefiore Hospital 3459-5th Avenue Pittsburgh, 15213	3	1
Presbyterian University Hospital Lothrop Street Pittsburgh, 15213	1	1
St. Francis General Hospital 45th Street at Penn Avenue Pittsburgh, 15201	2	1
South Side Hospital of Pittsburgh 20th and Jane Streets Pittsburgh, 15203	1	1
University of Pittsburgh Thackerary and O'Hara Streets Pittsburgh, 15213	3	1
The Western Pennsylvania Hospital 4800 Friendship Street Pittsburgh, 15224	1	1
PUERTO RICO		
University of Puerto Rico Medical Sciences Campus San Juan, 00905	3	3

Name and Location of Program	Length of Program (years)	Annual Openings
SOUTH CAROLINA		
Medical College of South Carolina 167 Ashley Avenue Charleston, 29401	3	2
TENNESSEE		
University of Tennessee Memorial Research Center and Hospital Alcoa Highway Knoxville, 37920	3	1
City of Memphis Hospital 860 Madison Avenue Memphis, 38103	3	2
University of Tennessee 62 Dunlap Street Memphis, 38103	3	2
Vanderbilt University Hospital 21st Avenue, S. Nashville, 37203	3	2-3
TEXAS		
Baylor University 800 Hall Street Dallas, 75226	3	1
Parkland Memorial Hospital 5201 Harry Hines Boulevard Dallas, 75235	3	4
John Peter Smith Hospital 1500 S. Main Street Fort Worth, 76104	3	1
University of Texas Medical Branch Hospitals 8th and Mechanic Streets Galveston, 77550	3	1
The University of Texas Dental Branch 6516 John Freeman Avenue Houston, 77025	3-4	3

Name and Location of Program	Length of Program (years)	Annual Openings
University of Texas Medical School at San Antonio and Affiliated Hospitals 7703 Floyd Curl Drive San Antonio, 78229	3	1
VIRGINIA		
Norfolk General Hospital 600 Gresham Drive Norfolk, 23507	1	1
Virginia Commonwealth University Health Science Division Richmond, 23219	3	3
WASHINGTON		
University of Washington Health Sciences Building Seattle, 98105	3	2
WEST VIRGINIA		
West Virginia University Medical Center Morgantown, 26506	3	1
Ohio Valley General Hospital 20th and Eoff Streets Wheeling, 26003	2	One Resident every other year.
Wheeling Hospital 109 Main Street Wheeling, 26003	1	1
WISCONSIN		
LaCrosse Lutheran-Gunderson Clinic 1910 South Avenue LaCrosse, 54601	3	1

Source: C. Bassett Brown, D.D.S., Benton Harbor, Michigan, 1970.

Appendix J

Report of Circumstances Surrounding the

Admission of an NDA Member into the ADA

PO Box 146
Columbus, Mississippi
January 27, 1969

Subject: Report of circumstances leading up to and surrounding the admission of one NDA member into membership in the ADA.

To: The National Dental Association
        Attention: Dr. James C. Wallace, President
                   Dr. C. O. Simpkins, Chairman, Civil Rights
                   Committee

Dear Colleagues:

August 29, 1966 was the date that I first applied for active membership in the American Dental Association. January 20, 1969 was the date that I was accepted into the membership of the Northeast District Dental Society, Mississippi Dental Association, and the American Dental Association. During the period between August 29, 1966 and the present date I have received numerous letters and some telephone calls from you, expressing concern and requesting information as to the status of my application. Some of your correspondence touched on the matter of possible reasons why some NDA members were having difficulty in receiving acceptance into the membership of the ADA. Most of these communications I have never answered for one or more of the following several reasons:

163

1. There had been no change in the status of my application.

2. I didn't want to make an evaluation that, even though true, might have become the basis for denial of membership.

3. Prior to the present time I didn't have sufficient clerical help to make a detailed written report.

First of all, let me say that I was not at all surprised when I was informed that I was accepted into membership of the American Dental Association on January 20, 1969. I say this because at no time did I lose faith in the majority of the people of Mississippi to do the right thing when the facts are known. The initial small opposition to my acceptance into ADA membership was based upon "hearsay" evidence and it was more than countermanded by numerous recommendations of approval from local people and others who knew the real facts. If I had thought that there would have been opposition to my original application I would have had letters of recommendation sent in 1966 instead of the latter part of 1968 and the first part of 1969. Dr. A. S. Thomas of Tupelo, Mississippi, not only did not receive any opposition but was invited to become a member of the Northeast District Dental Society in 1967. Dr. Thomas was most cooperative in helping to expedite favorable action on my application. I have recently been informed that Dr. Jones of Jackson, Mississippi has also been accepted into active membership of ADA.

In view of the great influence of the ADA in affecting the lives of all Americans and many others, I believe that membership in the ADA is not only a privilege but is also a duty of every dentist. From the moment that I found in 1950 that the recommendation of a member of the ADA was required in order to take the State Board of Dental Examination in Mississippi at that time, I knew the necessity of every dentist becoming a member of the ADA.

Although I don't believe that any Negro dentist in Mississippi will experience in the future any great difficulty in getting admitted into active membership in the ADA, I do believe that as long as there is one dentist of any race anywhere having difficulty that one of the following three things ought to be done immediately by the House of Delegates of the American Dental Association:

1. Permanently recall all requirements for admission into active ADA membership except the following:

   a. To be a graduate of an approved dental school.

   b. To be duly licensed to practice in the state where membership is being sought.

   c. To submit required application and annual dues.

2. The parent body of the American Dental Association should have a board of review with full authority to review and to reserve the actions of component and constituent societies in matters relating to membership.

3. For a period of five years next following the graduation of a dentist from dental school and/or from the date of the adoption of the ADA resolution, all requirements for acceptance into active membership into the American Dental Association should be suspended, except the following:

   a. To be a graduate of an approved dental school.

   b. To be duly licensed to practice in the state where membership is being sought.

   c. To submit the required application and annual dues.

The effect of this third proposed resolution should be to immediately give every ethical dentist an opportunity to become an active member of that body that is the official voice of dentistry in the United States of America. It will also give continued hope to those who seek responsible local control. The action should be welcomed by those who want to see all ethical dentists immediately accepted into membership in the ADA. So long as there are possible roadblocks to membership there will be many ethical dentists all over the United States who will never apply for membership in the ADA. To them rejection would be personally embarrassing.

I am certainly grateful to the NDA, the ADA, and to all of the people of my state who supported my application for membership into the American Dental Association. So many people made a contribution that I am unable to determine who or what did the most good. In order that you may make your own evaluation, I am attaching to this letter some of the pertinent correspondence in the case.

The following closing sentence was included in a letter to all of the dentists of my hometown in which I requested support of my application for active ADA membership:

"I assure you that when I am admitted into the membership I will do everything I can to maintain the high standards of the society and to be the type of member of which we all can be proud."

Respectfully yours,

E. J. Stringer, DDS

cc: The president-elect of the National Dental Association
The Mississippi Dental Society

May 18, 1966

Dr. Fayette Williams, Jr., Secretary
First District
The Mississippi Dental Association
Tupelo, Mississippi

Dear Dr. Williams:

Please send application blanks and other information that will be
needed by me in order to apply for membership in the American
Dental Association.

Yours truly,

E. J. Stringer, DDS

May 23, 1966

Dr. E. J. Stringer
PO Box 146
114½ Fourth Street, South
Columbus, Mississippi

Dear Dr. Stringer:

I forwarded your request for an application for membership in the
American Dental Society to our secretary, Dr. Jim Edwards of New
Albany.

Very sincerely yours,

Fayette Williams, Jr., DDS

Northeast Mississippi Dental
Society
Dr. James M. Edwards,
Secretary-Treasurer
Huston Building
New Albany, Mississippi
Friday, June 3, 1966

Dr. E. J. Stringer
Box 146
Columbus, Mississippi

Doctor:

Enclosed please find application for membership in American
Dental Association. This must be filled out completely and returned
to me any time before our next business meeting, the exact date of
which I'm not certain, but approximately January 20, 1967. Enclose
a check for dues if you wish.

$44.00	Mississippi Dental Association
40.00	American Dental Association
6.00	Northeast Dental Association

Total $90.00

It will not be necessary to enclose check; dues are delinquent after
March 31 and $10.00 fee is then assessed.

Respectfully,

James M. Edwards, DDS
Secretary-Treasurer

August 29, 1966

Name: E. J. Stringer, DDS
Address: PO Box 146, 114½ S. 4th Street
City: Columbus   State: Mississippi
Date of Birth: September 16, 1919
Graduate of: Meharry Medical College, Nashville, Tennessee
                    (Name of School)
License State of: Mississippi
Year of Graduation: 1950   Year of License: 1950
_____ Former Member   _____ New Member

If former member:
Period of Former Membership _____

If New Member:

I certify that I am an ethical practitioner of dentistry and hereby apply for active membership in:

Northeast Mississippi Dental Society
(Name of Component Society)

If elected to membership it is understood that I will become an active member of:

Mississippi Dental Association
(Name of Constituent Society)

I hereby apply for membership in the American Dental Association and state and local societies and enclose $90.00 as annual membership dues for one year to be apportioned as follows: Local Society $6.00, of which $_____ is for a subscription to _____ State Society $44.00, of which $_____ is for a subscription to _____ for one year. American Dental Association, $40.00 of which $3.50 is for a subscription to the *Journal* of the American Dental Association for one year. Total $90.00.

Application Received _____ Amount Received with application
_____   *(Date)*

Referred to Committee on Membership Admission _____
                                            (Date)

Approved _____ Disapproved _____

Committee on Membership Admissions:

_____   _____ Elected
Chairman

_____   _____ Rejected
_____

By action of _____
                    Name of Body Taking Action at the meeting held on

_____
                                    Date

Membership Card forwarded _____ *(Date)*

Secretary _____

Name of Society _____

September 15, 1966

Dr. William A. Garrett, President
The American Dental Association
Candler Building
Atlanta, Georgia

Dear Dr. Garrett:

I was happy to see you and to have the opportunity to talk with you
at the recent annual meeting of the National Dental Association in
New York City. As usual you were very effective in extending
greetings.

It is believed that you will be happy to know that I was invited to
and did attend a recent 2-day conference on Periodontics, Oral
Diagnosis and Oral Pathology at the University of Mississippi at
Oxford. The conference was sponsored by the Northeast Mississippi
Dental Society and was held August 31 and September 1, 1966. I
was very cordially received. Colonel Bkaskar of Walter Reed Army
Medical Center was the Clinician throughout the two days. The
applause that was given him at the conclusion of the Conference
was long and loud.

On August 29, 1966 I submitted my application for membership in
the Northeast Mississippi Dental Society. I am very proud of the
certificate that I received as a result of attending the recent dental
Conference and I do hope that my application for membership will
be approved at the next annual meeting of the Northeast Mississippi
Dental Society.

It is my hope that you will be able to accomplish most of your
objectives during the term of your office as President of the
American Dental Association. I am sure that no president ever does
all of the things that he would like to do during one term of office.

My wife joins me in extending best regards to Mrs. Garrett and to you.

Respectfully yours,

E. J. Stringer

2 Encls: General Information Bulletin and Registration List

Dr. William A. Garrett
President-Elect
833 Candler Building
Atlanta, Georgia 30303
September 29, 1966

Dear Dr. Stringer:

Have just returned from Honolulu where I attended the Hawaii State Dental Association. It was good to have your nice letter. I enjoyed being at your N.Y. meeting and visiting with you.

Am sure you profited by attending the Conference on Pathology. Dr. Bhaskar is an outstanding essayist. I always learn something when I have the privilege to hear him.

I trust and believe you will hear favorably from the Northeast Mississippi Dental Society.

Thank you for your good wishes during my year as President. My best regards to you and Mrs. Stringer.

Sincerely,

Wm. Garrett

MEMORANDUM

On January 20, 1967 I received a long distance telephone call from Dr. James Edwards, Secretary-Treasurer of the Northeast Mississippi Dental Society. The following is the substance of the telephone conversation between Dr. Edwards and me:

> Dr. Edwards said that my application for ADA membership was not approved during the January 1967 Annual Meeting of the Northeast District Dental Society. He wanted to know whether or not I wanted to have the $90.00 membership fee returned to me or to be kept by the Society while my application was being considered by the Judicial Committee of the Northeast Mississippi Dental Society. I told Dr. Edwards that I wanted the application and the $90.00 retained by the Society for consideration and that I wanted him to write me and tell me why my application had not been approved. He said that he was authorized to call me. He also said that the application was referred to the Judicial Committee for the purpose of clearing up some questions that could not be answered during the annual meeting. I told Dr. Edwards that I was quite willing to appear before any committee, anywhere at anytime. In reply to a question, Dr. Edwards said that three other applicants had been unanimously approved for membership during the January 1967 annual meeting and that one of the members was Dr. A. S. Thomas of Tupelo, Mississippi.

E. J. Stringer

MEMORANDUM

About 1:30 p.m., Friday, January 9, 1968, I made a long distance telephone call to Dr. James Edwards of New Albany, Mississippi. The following is the substance of the telephone conversation between Dr. James M. Edwards, Secretary-Treasurer of New Albany, Mississippi, of Northeast Mississippi Dental Society, and myself;

Operator:	Long distance is calling Dr. Edwards.
Dental Assistant:	Who is calling please?
Operator:	Dr. Stringer of Columbus, Missis-sippi.
Dental Assistant:	Dr. Edwards is coming in right now.
Dr. Edwards:	Hello.
Dr. Stringer:	Dr. Edwards, this is Dr. Stringer of Columbus. How are you?
Dr. Edwards:	All right. (Sounded friendly)
Dr. Stringer:	Dr. Edwards, I have not received my membership card for ADA. What is the status of my application?
Dr. Edwards:	I returned your $90.00 this morning. I have the report of the Judicial Committee right here. I will read it: "We, the members of the Judicial Committee, hereby report that Dr. E. J. Stringer of Columbus, Mississippi, does not meet the requirements for membership in the 1st District Dental Society. This recommendation is based upon reports from: a. The Mississippi State Sovereignty Committee b. The Credit Bureau c. Various character witnesses."
Dr. Stringer:	Doctor, I am sorry that I did not get to appear before the Judicial Committee. What do you suggest that I should do now?
Dr. Edwards:	I would just follow the leads. In view of the report of the Judicial Committee, I didn't know anything to do except to return your money.

Dr. Stringer:	Thank you very much for your courtesy. Goodbye.
Dr. Edwards:	Goodbye.

E. J. Stringer

PO Box 146
Columbus, Mississippi
October 22, 1968

Dr. James C. Wallace, President
The National Dental Association
3600 W. 16th Street
Chicago, Illinois

Dear Dr. Wallace:

It is a genuine pleasure to address you as "Mr. President." In the entire history of the National Dental Association, there probably has been no person who has been more deserving than you to hold the organization's highest office. I wish for you a most successful administration.

I regret very much that for the first time in many many years, I was unable to attend the recent meeting of the NDA. About the time of the annual meeting in Houston I was a patient in the Baptist Memorial Hospital in Memphis, Tennessee. Following a period of very intensive examinations I was given a clean bill of health except for fungus infection of the feet, of which I am now being treated. My physician emphasized the necessity of one day of complete rest each week.

In your recent letter you asked two questions concerning my application for membership in the ADA: (a) if I applied for membership in 1968? (b) if so, what specifically happened?

In August 1966, I submitted my application and cashier's check for $90.00 to the Secretary of the Northeast Mississippi District Dental Society.

In January 1967, I received a telephone call from the Secretary of the Northeast Mississippi District Dental Society saying that the application had been referred to the Judicial Committee of the Northeast Mississippi District Dental Society.

February 9, 1968, I called the Secretary of the Northeast District Dental Society and inquired about the status of my membership. He informed me that the above-mentioned Committee had made its report and that in the opinion of the Committee as adopted by the membership, I was not qualified to become a member of the ADA at that time. The Secretary also stated that the report from the Committee was based on three things:

a. A report from the sovereignty Committee of the State of Mississippi,

b. Local character witnesses; and,

c. The Columbus, Mississippi Credit Bureau.

On February 10, 1968, I received a personal check in the amount of $90.00 from the Secretary of the Northeast Mississippi District Dental Society, representing a refund to me of membership fees (Local, State and National) previously submitted by me by cashier's check in August 1966.

I intend to resubmit an application prior to the January 1969 meeting of the Northeast Mississippi District Dental Society.

I have several suggestions to make regarding the business of active membership in the ADA:

a. In my opinion, every dentist who is a graduate of an approved dental school and who is licensed to practice in a state should be automatically accepted into the local, state and national organizations on the basis of application and dues only.

b. If the parent body of ADA does not presently share the philosophy as expressed in item above, I can see only one other reasonable alternative and that is for the parent body to set up a Board of Review and if necessary to reverse the actions of the local and state organizations in regard to actions relating to membership.

c. If the parent body of ADA is not willing to measure up to its responsibility to all of its citizens at this time, it is believed that deprived citizens will have no choice except to seek relief through the courts.

Yours truly,

E. J. Stringer, DDS
Box 146
Columbus, Mississippi

PO Box 146
Columbus, Mississippi
November, 1968

Dr. Frank C. Baker
Secretary-Treasurer
Northeast District Dental Society
810 Garfield
Tupelo, Mississippi

Dear Dr. Baker:

Please send application blanks and other information that will be needed by me in order to apply for membership in the American Dental Association.

Sincerely,

E. J. Stringer, DDS

Frank C. Baker, DDS
810 Garfield
Tupelo, Mississippi 38801
December 4, 1968

Dr. E. J. Stringer
PO Box 146
Columbus, Mississippi

Dear Dr. Stringer:

Enclosed is an application blank for membership in the Northeast District Dental Society, Mississippi Dental Association, and the American Dental Association.

The total amount of membership fee is still not definite because of the increase in American Dental Association dues approved by the House of Delegates of the American Dental Association last month in Miami.

Sincerely,

Frank C. Baker, DDS
Secretary-Treasurer
Northeast District Dental
    Society

Dr. E. J. Stringer, Dentist
PO Box 146
114½ Fourth Street, South
Columbus, Mississippi 39701

Dr. Frank C. Baker, Secretary-Treasurer
Northeast District Dental Society
810 Garfield
Tupelo, Mississippi 38801

Dear Dr. Baker:

On August 29, 1966 I applied for membership in the American
Dental Association by submitting to the Secretary-Treasurer of the
Northeast Mississippi Dental Society an accomplished application
form and a bank money order in the amount of $90.00.

On or about February 1, 1967 I talked by telephone with the
Secretary-Treasurer of the Northeast Mississippi Dental Society,
during which time he indicated that my application was being
referred to a committee to investigate certain questions that could
not be cleared up during the annual meeting in January 1967.

On February 9, 1968 I talked again by telephone with Dr. James M.
Edwards of New Albany. He informed me that he had returned to
me on February 9, 1968 the $90.00 that was sent to him on August
1966. Dr. Edwards also read to me that part of the report of the
Judiciary Committee which said in substance that I did not meet the
requirements for membership in the 1st District Dental Society and
that the report was based upon reports received from the
Sovereignty Committee of the State of Mississippi, the Credit
Bureau and various character witnesses.

On February 10, 1968 I received in the mail a check from Dr.
Edwards in the amount of $90.00.

For the following reasons I am hereby submitting another
application for membership and a cashier's check in the amount of
$105.00.

   1. I do know that I am an ethical dentist, a reputable practitioner,

a qualified Doctor of Dental Surgery, a graduate of an accredited dental school, and fully licensed to practice in the State of Mississippi.

2. It is my opinion that it is a duty as well as a privilege for every member of a given profession to become a member of that professional organization that is the official organ of that profession. The American Dental Association is without a doubt the official voice of Dentistry in the United States of America.

3. It is believed that those who may have made unfavorable statements about me were not deliberately trying to discredit me but were merely expressing what they had heard or what they had read rather than what they personally knew.

4. It is believed that the members of the Northeast Mississippi Dental Society would not knowingly deny membership to any qualified applicant.

5. With regard to anything that might have been said by the State Sovereignty Committee I can only say that I do not deny that I am of the opinion that segregation based upon race, creed, color or previous condition of servitude is not only legally but morally wrong.

6. With regard to the testimony of certain above mentioned character witnesses, I hereby submit at this time the names of the following persons, all of whom I believe will testify that to the best of their knowledge and belief that I am a person of excellent character and reputation:

Dr. William Garrett
Past President
The American Dental
    Association
Candler Building
Atlanta, Georgia

R. W. Harrison, DDS
President
The North Mississippi Medical,
    Dental and Pharmaceutical
    and Nurses Society
Yazoo City, Mississippi

Justice Thurgood Marshall
Member
The United States Supreme
    Court
Supreme Court Building
Washington, D.C.

Mr. Jesse Elkin
President
Columbus-Lowndes Chamber of
    Commerce
Waters Building
Columbus, Mississippi

Rev. Mark Kuehnert
President
The United Ministerial
  Association of Lowndes
  County
1211-18th Avenue North
Columbus, Mississippi

Mr. William H. Walker
Manager
Mississippi State Employment
  Service
Columbus, Mississippi

Dr. J. C. Wallace
President
The National Dental Association
3600 W. 16th Street
Chicago, Illinois

The Honorable Robert Harmon
Mayor
The City of Columbus
Columbus, Mississippi

Dr. L. T. Britton
President
The Mississippi Dental Society
Greenville, Mississippi

Mr. Ben Owen
Attorney-at-law
Representative from Lowndes
  County
Mississippi House of
  Representatives
Columbus, Mississippi

Senator William G. Burgin
Attorney-at-law
Member of the Mississippi
  Senate
Columbus, Mississippi

Lieutenant Colonel A. N.
  Temple
United States Air Force
  (Retired)
Route 4, Box 363
Columbus, Mississippi

Dr. James I. Califf
Director
The Reading Center, MSCW
Columbus, Mississippi

A. S. Thomas, DDS
Tupelo, Mississippi

Mr. H. K. Van Every
Attorney-at-law
Columbus, Mississippi

Mr. A. Y. Banks
Postmaster
Columbus, Mississippi

Rev. W. M. Redmond
District Superintendent
United Methodist Church
Member of the Oxford City
  School Board
Oxford, Mississippi

Autrey Presley, DDS
Holly Springs, Mississippi

Mr. M. C. Edwards
Sheriff
Lowndes County
Columbus, Mississippi

G. C. Welch, DDS
Columbus, Mississippi

Rev. Hunt Comer
Minister
St. Paul Episcopal Church
Columbus, Mississippi

Mr. Shield Sims
Attorney-at-law
Vice President
The Columbus-Lowndes
    Chamber of Commerce
Columbus, Mississippi

7. With regard to the report of the Credit Bureau, I have not been told what it says. I don't claim to have the highest credit rating with Dun and Bradstreet, and neither am I a dentist who possesses great economic security. I have tried during the past 18 years to become involved in a responsible way with community growth and development. Specifically, I have served as president of three of our most responsible and influential local organizations:

The Columbus Branch of the National Association for the
Advancement of Colored People.

The Lowndes County League of Registered Voters.

The Lowndes County Area Headstart Program.

There have been those who, for various reasons, have opposed the purposes of these organizations and have therefore opposed me as president and have used various means to try to discredit me. One of these means apparently has been application of economic pressure which obviously would make it difficult to always pay everything by the 10th of each month. If not by the 10th, I usually have gotten there before the end of the month. The person who is in a position to know most about my present credit standing is the President of the local bank with which I transact my business. I respectfully suggest that you will contact Mr. John R. Henry, President of the Merchants and Farmers Bank, Columbus, Mississippi.

8. Because of the long delay involved in the consideration of my application of the Northeast Mississippi Dental Society, and in view of my present statement, it is believed that the members of Northeast Mississippi Dental Society would want me to appear before the Membership Committee and/or the parent body not later than the date of the next annual meeting of the Society in January 1969. For the purpose of further clarification I am hereby requesting that I will have an opportunity to be heard and that any necessary investigation will be made prior to or during the annual meeting of

the Society in January 1969 so that there will be no further delay regarding my acceptance into the membership of the American Dental Association.

I assure you that when I am admitted into the membership I will do everything that I can do to maintain the high standards of the Society and to be the type of member of which we all can be proud.

Respectfully yours,

E. J. Stringer, DDS

2 Enclosures
   Accomplished Application Form
   Cashier's Check
   (Local and State Dues, including subscription for *Journal* of Mississippi Dental Association) $50.00
   (National Dues-ADA, including subscription for ADA *Journal*) $55.00   Total: $105.00

Sample Letter Written By Dr. Stringer Requesting A Character Reference

December 26, 1978

Mr. John R. Henry
President
The Merchants and Farmers Bank
111 Fifth Street, South
Columbus, Mississippi

Dear Mr. Henry:

I have applied for membership in the District, State and National bodies of the American Dental Association, the official voice of organized dentistry in the United States of America.

In order to have my application favorably considered, it is necessary for me to have several individuals from Columbus to express their opinions as to my character and also my reputation in the community. I would be very grateful if you would send a letter of recommendation to: Dr. Frank C. Baker, Secretary-Treasurer, Northeast District Dental Society, 810 Garfield, Tupelo, Mississippi 38801.

In your letter to Dr. Baker it would be helpful if you would also mention that I am in good standing with the Merchants and Farmers Bank.

Yours truly,

E. J. Stringer, DDS

Letter of Reference

December 26, 1968

Dr. Frank C. Baker
Secretary-Treasurer
Northeast District Dental Society
810 Garfield
Tupelo, Mississippi 38801

Dear Dr. Baker:

It is our understanding that E. J. Stringer, DDS, is applying for
membership in the District, State, and National Groups of the
American Dental Association.

Dr. Stringer has requested that I address you in this connection, and
I am pleased to recommend him.

Dr. Stringer is a leader among his people in the Columbus area, and,
to the best of my knowledge, he represents a constructive rather
than a radical type of citizenship.

Every indication that we have had shows him to be a man of
excellent character, and in the handling of his personal business
affairs here at the bank, he enjoys a good reputation.

I trust that your professional group will extend Dr. Stringer fullest
consideration for membership.

Sincerely yours,

John R. Henry, President

cc: Dr. E. J. Stringer

MEMORANDUM

On or about December 24, 1968, I received a long distance telephone call from Dr. Robert E. Mathis of Corinth, Mississippi who identified himself as Chairman of the Membership Committee of the Northeast Mississippi District Dental Society. The following is the substance of the telephone conversation between Dr. Mathis and me:

> After identifying himself, Dr. Mathis expressed the hope that I would not become offended by anything that he might say or ask. I assured him that I don't have a chip on my shoulder, neither am I easily offended. He asked if I knew the reason or reasons why my previous application for ADA membership had not been approved. I repeated to him what had been told me by the Secretary of the ADA component. I repeated to him my opposition to segregation based upon race, creed, color or previous condition of servitude. Dr. Mathis assured me that as far as he was concerned no one would be denied ADA membership because of race or personal views. He also said that, prior to the time of action by the body, I would be notified of the recommendation of the Membership Committee.

E. J. Stringer

January 2, 1969

Dr. Frank C. Baker
Secretary-Treasurer
Northeast District Dental Society
810 Garfield Street
Tupelo, Mississippi 38801

Dear Dr. Baker:

I am writing you this letter in regards to the character and
reputation of Dr. E. J. Stringer, who I understand has an application
to become a member of the Northeast District Dental Society.

I have personally known Dr. Stringer for the past two years. He is
an active member of the Columbus-Lowndes Chamber of Commerce
and, in my opinion, a leader in our community. In my dealings with
Dr. Stringer, he has always been fair, courteous, and most
important, honest. I would be glad to recommend Dr. Stringer for
membership.

Sincerely,

W. B. James
Justice of the Peace, District II

January 7, 1969

Mr. John R. Henry
President
Merchants and Farmers Bank
111 S. 5th Street
Columbus, Mississippi 39701

Dear Mr. Henry:

Thank you very much for the letter of recommendation that you were kind enough to send in support of my application for membership in the American Dental Association.

Yours truly,

E. J. Stringer, DDS

January 7, 1969

Mr. Samuel A. Pope
Chief of Police
Columbus, Mississippi 39701

Dear Mr. Pope:

Thank you very much for the letter of recommendation that you
were kind enough to send in support of my application for
membership in the American Dental Association.

Yours truly,

E. J. Stringer, DDS

January 8, 1969

Attorney Ben Owen
Representative from Lowndes County
Mississippi House of Representatives
508 2nd Avenue North
Columbus, Mississippi 39701

Dear Lawyer Owen:

Thank you very much for the letter of recommendation that you
were kind enough to send in support of my application for
membership in the American Dental Association.

Yours truly,

E. J. Stringer

American Dental Association
211 East Chicago Avenue
Chicago, Illinois

January 8, 1969

Dr. James C. Wallace, Jr.
President
National Dental Association
3600 West 16th Street
Chicago, Illinois 60623

Dear Doctor Wallace:

As mentioned in our telephone conversation this evening, I am enclosing for your information copies of Dr. Hillenbrand's letters requesting the reasons for rejection of the previous membership application of Drs. Carline, Martin, and Stringer.

Cordially,

Howard I. Wells, Jr.
Consultant, Office of the
Executive Director

cc: Dr. Harold Hillenbrand, Mr. P. Goulding
Dr. Bernard J. Conway, Mr. J. P. Noone

American Dental Association
211 East Chicago Avenue
Chicago, Illinois
January 8, 1969

Dr. Frank C. Baker
Secretary
Northeast Mississippi Dental Society
Tupelo, Mississippi

Dear Doctor Baker:

We have received a copy of a letter which Dr. E. J. Stringer of
Columbus, Mississippi wrote to the President of the National Dental
Association. The letter was in reply to a request for information
concerning alleged discrimination on entrance into membership in
constituent and component societies of the American Dental
Association.

Dr. Stringer stated that his application for membership in the
Northeast Mississippi Dental District Society had not been accepted
and that he intended to resubmit his application prior to the January
1969 meeting of the Society.

At the request of the Board of Trustees I would appreciate receiving
from you a statement of the reason or reasons for the Society's
rejection of Dr. Stringer's previous membership application.

Cordially,

Harold Hillenbrand, DDS
Executive Director

cc: Dr. Robert E. Mathis
Dr. Fayette C. Williams, Jr.
Dr. David M. Miller
Mr. Jerry Bagley
Dr. Arthur W. Kellner

A. S. Thomas
416 North Spring Street
Tupelo, Mississippi
January 13, 1969

Dear Dr. Stringer:

I talked with Dr. Baker today to find out how everything was shaping up. He said the Judicial Committee met yesterday, January 12, 1969 and discussed your case . . .

Do all you can to get your hometown dentists to speak for you. Dr. Baker said he wrote you or was going to do so.

Yours truly,

A. S. Thomas, DDS

January 13, 1969

Dr. E. J. Stringer
PO Box 146
Columbus, Mississippi

Dear Dr. Stringer:

Your application has been reviewed by the Judicial Committee of the Northeast Mississippi Dental Society. Your application, along with the others received, will be submitted to the general membership of the Northeast Mississippi Dental Society for their consideration during the business session at the annual meeting next Monday, January 20, 1969.

Sincerely,

Frank C. Baker, DDS
Secretary-Treasurer
Northeast Mississippi Dental
    Society

January 11, 1969

Dr. E. J. Stringer
PO Box 146
Columbus, Mississippi

Dear Dr. Stringer:

We presented your case to the ADA at their recent session in Miami,
and during the meeting, and will followup on it in Chicago,
February 3, 1969 at our conference with ADA officials. Will it be
possible for you to come up and bring your case in person? Rest
assured that we are doing everything possible, and I am confident
that we are going to get the same favorable results for you as we
were able to get for Dr. Kilgore from Johnson City, Tennessee.

If you know of any other dentist in your state experiencing similar
problems, kindly let me hear from you giving names and addresses,
as well as any other pertinent information, as soon as possible.
Expecting to hear from you soon, I am

Very truly yours,

James C. Wallace, Jr., DDS
President

cc: NDA Officers
Dr. Simpkins
Dr. Adams

PO Box 146
Columbus, Mississippi
January 14, 1969

Subject: Request for Endorsement of Membership Application

To: The Dentists of Columbus, Mississippi

Dear Colleague(s):

This letter is to ask for your support of my application for active membership into the Northeast District Dental Society. I sincerely hope and believe that the application will be favorably considered during the January 1969 meeting of the Northeast District Dental Society. You probably already know that one of my dental school classmates, Dr. A. S. Thomas of Tupelo, became a member of the Northeast District Dental Society in January 1968.

In 1950 it was necessary for me to receive the recommendation of a member of the American Dental Association in order to take the State Board Dental Examination. I was fortunate to be able to receive that recommendation from the late Dr. George Dowdle of Columbus and his name now appears on my dental license. Because of Dr. Dowdle's faith in me, because of my personal love for the profession, and because of the realization of the great need for dentists in this area, I have tried during the past 18 years to maintain a high standard of dental excellence.

I am now coming to you in 1969 asking you to help me to become a member of that organization that is the official voice of dentistry in the United States of America. You certainly know much better than I of many of the benefits and meaning of membership in the American Dental Association.

When my application for membership comes before the body for consideration I certainly hope that you will vote that I will be accepted into the membership. If there are any questions relating to me I would be very happy to have the opportunity to talk with you at a time and place that will be convenient for you.

I assure you that when I am admitted into the membership I will do everything that I can to maintain the high standards of the Society and to be the type of member of which we all can be proud.

Respectfully yours,

E. J. Stringer, DDS

January 22, 1969

Dr. E. J. Stringer
PO Box 146
Columbus, Mississippi 39701

Dear Dr. Stringer:

Your application for membership has been approved by the general membership of the Northeast District Dental Society. I am enclosing your membership card for this year, 1969.

Sincerely,

Frank C. Baker, DDS
Northeast Mississippi Dental
Society

January 25, 1969

Subject: Expression of Gratitude

To: The Dentists of Columbus, Mississippi

Dear Colleague(s):

Thank you very much for your support of my application for active membership into the American Dental Association.

Respectfully yours,

E. J. Stringer, DDS

January 14, 1969

James C. Wallace, Jr.
President
National Dental Association, Inc.
3600 West 16th Street
Chicago, Illinois 60623

Dear Dr. Wallace:

Received your letter of January 11th requesting the names of
persons having problems to become members of the American
Dental Association.

I submit that every black dentist that is not now a member of the
American Dental Association in the South, even where others have
been accepted, is receiving difficulty and having problems. They are
having problems because:

   Number one, they have seen and heard of the problems of
acceptance of their fellow black practitioner upon his plight to enter
into the mainstream of dentistry;
   Number two, some have not seen or been stimulated into the
realization of the need of becoming members of the American
Dental Association;
   Number three, others would not want to jeopardize their minority
positions in a small town by applying for membership; and,
   Number four, others have expressed extreme difficulty in securing
necessary sponsors, or do not have the social contact with the white
practitioner to request his sponsorship.

Therefore, we should not require of our membership any other
burdens than they already have. We should relieve them of any
burden of proof, sponsorship, photographs, and other subterfuge
that is not required of the white practitioner. When and only when
these roadblocks are removed from the top and the American Dental
Association itself "stops playing games" and removes all of these
barriers can we say that we have completed our mission to end
discrimination in dentistry. *There is no victory until we have been
victorious!*

Enclosed is the report of the Chairman of the Civil Rights Committee. Shall be contacting you within a few days as to the possibility of my being in Chicago for the midwinter meeting and participation in the Subcommittee of the Liaison Committee on Civil Rights. With every best wish,

Sincerely,

C. O. Simpkins, DDS
Chairman
Civil Rights Committee

Bibliography

Bronson, Fred, and Howard Hall. "Black Dentistry in Cincinnati." Paper prepared for *Profile of the Negro in American Dentistry*.

Culp, D. W., ed. *Twentieth Century Negro Literature*. Atlanta: J. L. Nicols Co., 1902.

Dummett, Clifton O. "Chronological Sequence of Events Relating to Dentistry in the Afro-American Population: 1963-70." NDA *Quarterly* 28 (1970): 42.

——————. "A Chronology Updated: Recent Events in the Negro's Advancement in Dentistry in the United States." NDA *Quarterly* 21 (1963): 147.

——————. "Dentistry as a Career for Women." Brochure prepared for Meharry Medical College School of Dentistry, 1945.

——————. *Growth and Development of the Negro in Dentistry in the United States*. Chicago: The Stanek Press, 1952.

Freese, Arthur S. "6000 Years of Dentistry." *CAL* Magazine, October 1966, p. 18.

Graber, T. M. *Orthodontics, Principles and Practice*, 2d rev. ed. Philadelphia: W. B. Saunders, Co., 1968.

Henry, Joseph L. "Bridging the Gap." *Journal of Dental Education*, January 1971.

"Historical Background of Lincoln Dental Society." Lincoln Dental Society *Bulletin* 27 (1970): 6-11.

Lee, Ulysses. "The Employment of Negro Troops." Office of the Chief of Military History, United States Army. Washington, D.C., 1966.

Lentchner, Emil W. "Discrimination in the Dental Profession." NDA *Quarterly* 25 (1966): 9-12.

Lewis, Richard A. "U.S. Dentists: Distribution in Relation to Population." *JADA* 82 (1971): 480.

Linn, Erwin L. "Black Dentists: Some Circumstances about Their Occupational Choice." *Journal of Dental Education*, March 1972.

Moyers, R. E. *Handbook of Orthodontics*. 2d rev. ed. Chicago: Medical Publishers, 1963.

Old Dominion Dental Society, Norfolk. "History of Negro Dentists in Virginia."

Sarner, Harvey. *Dental Jurisprudence*. Tampa, Florida: W. F. Poe, 1963.

Simpkins, C. O. "Report of Civil Rights Committee." Minutes of Executive Board and General Session of the NDA, August 1966.

Sinks, Robert M. *A Brief History of Dentistry*. Dallas, Texas: Gallery Collections, 1971.

Stampp, Kenneth M. *The Peculiar Institution*. New York: Alfred A. Knopf, 1956.

Stout, Walter C. *The First Hundred Years in Dentistry in Texas*. Dallas, Texas: The Eagan Company, 1969.

Thompson, Robert. "Considerations Involving the Shortage of Black Dentists." *Journal of Dental Education*, December 1970, pp. 82-88.

Index

Accreditation of dental schools, 18, 23, 125

Adams (Dr.), 194

Advertising by dentists, 14; 15

Alabama: Birmingham, 42, 60; Huntsville, 63, 65; University of, 87

Alabama Dental Hygienists' Association, 54

Allen, Millison, 12

Allen, William H., 21, 42

Alpha Phi Alpha fraternity, 26

Altemus, Leonard, 40

American Association of Dental Examiners, 101, 103

American Association of Dental Schools, 25

American Association of Endodontists, 34

American Board of Dental Public Health, 33

American Board of Oral Pathology, 35

American Board of Orthodontics, 40

American Board of Prosthodontics, 43

American Dental Assistants Association, 53

American Dental Association (ADA), 11, 25, 56, 71, 73, 80-92, 163-199; American Fund for Dental Education of, 25; American Fund for Dental Health of, 25, 37, 56, 138; black dentists in, 76-77, 80-93, 163-199; Bureau of Economics, Research, and Statistics of, 42; cases against, 83-84, 87-88; Council on Dental Education of, 18, 23, 44, 135; dental specialties recognized by, 30-31; discriminatory practices of constituent societies, 81-84, 88, 89, 92, 163-199; Division of Educational Measurement of, 28, 124; *Journal*, 81, 82, 83, 86, 87; membership requirements, 80-81; nondiscriminatory resolutions of, 81-82, 90

American Dental Trade Association: Student Loan Fund, 138

American Public Health Association, 41

American Society of Oral Surgery, 36

American University (Beirut, Lebanon), 21

Ancient Egyptian Arabic Order of Nobles of the Mystic Shrine, 26

Anderson, Arnett A., 101

Anderson, J.W., 20

The Annual Survey of Dental Educational Institutions (ADA), 124

Atlanta Constitution (Georgia), 83

Atlanta University, 60

Authors, list of contributing, 109